CARDIO CURES

Alternative Strategies for a Healthy Heart

Gary Bushkin, Ph.D., C.N.C., &
Estitta Bushkin, Ph.D., C.N.C.

Keats Publishing

Chicago   New York   San Francisco   Lisbon   London   Madrid   Mexico City
Milan   New Delhi   San Juan   Seoul   Singapore   Sydney   Toronto

Library of Congress Cataloging-in-Publication Data

Bushkin, Gary.
    Cardio cures : alternative strategies for a healthy heart / Gary Bushkin, Estitta
Bushkin.
        p.   cm.
    Includes bibliographical references and index.
    ISBN 0-658-01531-1 (alk. paper)
    1. Heart—Diseases—Popular works.   I. Bushkin, Estitta.   II. Title.

RC672 .B87   2001
616.1'2—dc21   2001038352

Keats Publishing

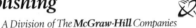

*A Division of The **McGraw·Hill** Companies*

1 2 3 4 5 6 7 8 9 0 DOC/DOC 0 9 8 7 6 5 4 3 2 1

ISBN 0-658-01531-1

This book was set in Monotype Garamond
Printed and bound by R. R. Donnelley—Crawfordsville

Cover design by Mike Stromberg/The Great American Art Co.
Interior design by Andrea Reider

McGraw-Hill books are available at special quantity discounts to use as premiums and
sales promotions, or for use in corporate training programs. For more information, please
write to the Director of Special Sales, Professional Publishing, McGraw-Hill, Two Penn
Plaza, New York, NY 10121-2298. Or contact your local bookstore.

Contents

Foreword

IN LATE SUMMER OF 1983, MY FATHER, MORRIS BUSHKIN, WAS victimized by a debilitating stroke that came without warning and dramatically changed forever the quality of his life, and the lives of close family members. He was only fifty-nine years old. Over the next nine years, his steady and unrelenting deterioration was both physically and emotionally distressing for everyone concerned. Then, in 1992, to further complicate his deteriorating health, he was diagnosed with cancer of the larynx. This stripped away his ability to communicate freely with the world. He was unable to speak without a cumbersome device, a microphone-shaped device that was held against the larynx to pick up vibrations of the vocal cords. Angry, depressed, and confined to a wheelchair, his life energy and desire to live ebbed rapidly. With little surprise, he left us quietly in 1995, barely seventy-two years old. We were deeply saddened by his years of worsening illness and declining health. Quite dismayed by how little traditional medical treatment had to offer him, Estitta and I became passionately inspired to seek the truth about the real causes of cardiovascular disease. We are still on the journey, but we have discovered and learned much that everyone should know.

Traditional Good-Spirited Naïveté and Confusion

For the most part, medical doctors and the medical community mean well. But, from the early days in medical school through internship and working in a practice, clinic, or hospital setting, their training leads them down a not-so-rosy path. It is a narrow path filled with good-spirited intentions and well-intended naïveté. Regrettably, for most of us, the training is lacking a scientifically and medically correct understanding of human metabolism and biochemistry, as well as the essential, critical role nutrition plays in the maintenance of optimum wellness. Despite the overwhelming amount of evidence to support the cause, philosophy, principles, and proven applications of natural medicine, many medical professionals continue to blindly plod along the path of quick, impersonal visits with patients. Meanwhile, high-pressure drug company representatives push new drugs that may kill you (Rezulin, Fen-Phen). Many doctors don't take the time or feel they have the time to learn and understand the true root causes of disease and illness, instead choosing the easier, more financially rewarding path of diagnose and prescribe, cut-and-burn medicine. In this mind-set, we cannot ever cure disease and illness but merely try to soften the blow by making it less painful, mentally and physically. It is the practice of suppression, both of knowledge and pain, a philosophy and style of practice we don't at all agree with.

Cardio Cures explores the groundbreaking cardiovascular scientific research of two-time Nobel Prize winner Linus Pauling, Ph.D., and world-renowned cardiologists and researchers Matthias Rath, M.D., Kilmer S. McCully, M.D., and Edward N. Siguel, M.D. We will also look closely at the research and written works of other prominent health professionals, along with the research insights and knowledge we have gained researching this book. So listen carefully. Cholesterol does not cause heart disease. This book is all about what does.

Cardio Cures will illustrate that chronic vitamin C deficiency, elevated lipoprotein(a), homocysteine, insulin, glucose, adrenalin, chronic systemic arterial inflammation, and C-reactive protein in the blood are primary independent risk factors and risk markers for heart disease that are far more significant than cholesterol is or ever will be.

Acknowledgments

WRITING THIS BOOK WAS A COMPLICATED PROCESS FOR US. We spent hundreds of hours conducting research, compiling information and data, reviewing scientific studies, drafting chapters, and making endless revisions. After going through reams of computer paper, we have finally arrived at what we sincerely believe is a thorough, accurate, and life-saving treatise on cardiovascular disease—America's number one killer.

Obviously, we could not, nor did we do it alone. The usually thankless job of assisting us in our efforts to educate the public in an accurate and thorough manner should be duly acknowledged. To all of you—the professionals, scientists, doctors, educators, colleagues, editors, librarians, and friends who gave your unselfish assistance, discussion, and interview time on the phone, via E-mail, and in person, we truly thank you.

To my father, whose miserable existence as a stroke and cancer victim ultimately created an overwhelming desire within us to uncover the truth about heart disease, this book is a constant reminder of your loving memory.

Disclaimer

THE HEALTH AND WELLNESS EDUCATION PRESENTED IN THIS book is not to be considered medical advice. It is provided solely for educational purposes as a comprehensive yet practical collection of nutrition, fitness, lifestyle, scientific, and medical information, and our own long-term personal experiences and applications that readers can consider in conjunction with advice from a qualified health practitioner.

Recommendations, suggestions, and references to food, nutritional supplements, exercise, stress management techniques, and our own personal experiences are offered only for education on how to build personal optimum cardiovascular and whole-body wellness and are not a promise or guarantee of results. No representations, whether expressed or implied, are made or given regarding the health or medical consequences of opinions contained in this book.

The authors and publisher assume no responsibility for any and all uses of the information in this book that may be used anytime by its readers. If you now have, or have had, medical, physical, or psychological problems of any kind in the past, or if you currently take prescription medications or receive physical or psychological therapies, the unapproved use of the information contained in this book is not recommended.

Introduction

MOST PEOPLE ARE CONFUSED ABOUT WHAT CAUSES A DISEASE, condition, or syndrome. With cardiovascular disease it is vitally important for us to make a clear distinction here between the causes and the effects. A good example of cause and effect takes us back to childhood days: A boy with a baseball throws the ball through a neighbor's window. What happens? The window shatters. Why? The force of the ball striking the window causes the window to shatter. The effect, or result, is a broken window. And so it is with cardiovascular disease. Unadulterated natural cholesterol produced by your liver, lipoprotein(a), cholesterol, and fats consumed in your food do not independently irritate the endothelial cells that protect artery linings. Nor do they damage the linings of your arteries. Rather, they arrive at the scene of arterial injury to repair the damage that has already been done. When they land at the site of an injury (lesion), they readily stick to the artery wall as a way of repairing the damage. After the repair is made they do not return from where they originated but remain at the site. Then they attract more of the same repair molecules and other undesirable biomolecules. As the quantity and size of these molecules increase, they begin to close off the artery, eventually blocking it, causing painful reduced blood flow (angina), a heart attack, or stroke.

The initial cause of the problem is chronic vitamin C deficiency, along with insufficient amounts of the amino acids lysine and proline. This leads to incorrect, structurally defective and insufficient production of collagen. Low collagen levels, lack of collagen, or collagen that is structurally defective causes arteries to become weak, thin, porous, inelastic, and inflexible. This subjects them to biochemical assaults from cardioirritants such as free radicals, homocysteine, glucose, insulin, adrenalin, cortisol, and physiological assaults from high blood pressure. The absence of Essential Fatty Acids (EFAs) leaves cell membranes permeable to toxins, restricts entry of nutrients and oxygen, prevents the elimination of toxins and metabolic wastes, and causes hardening of the cell membranes. Cells weaken and become exposed to injury. Cholesterol and lipoprotein(a) are not the cause of the problem; they are the body's preprogrammed metabolic responses to it. Their buildup eventually becomes a secondary cause of arteriosclerosis (thickening or hardening of the arteries) and atherosclerosis (fatty deposits in the arteries).

Congratulations! You are a member of the 50/50 club! First the bad news. You've got a 50/50 chance of developing heart disease! Now the good news. You can prevent it!

The Frightening Statistics

Consider these frightening facts:

- Cardiovascular disease (diseases of the heart and cardiovascular system, including coronary artery disease—CAD) is America's number one killer!
- About one out of every two people in the United States will die of some form of heart disease. Half the men and women just like you die of cardiovascular disease in the United States and other countries.
- Every thirty-three seconds, an American dies of heart disease.
- Over one million people in the United States die of cardiovascular disease each year.
- The World Health Organization tells us that cardiovascular disease is the cause of over twelve million deaths each year worldwide.

According to the American Heart Association:

- Nearly fifty-nine million Americans have some form of cardiovascular disease.
- Over one hundred million Americans are currently at risk.
- About two and a half million people suffer from angina.
- Nearly one and a half million people have a heart attack each year.
- Over five hundred thousand of those that have heart attacks are overweight.[1]
- There are more than twenty million reported cases of heart disease annually.
- Heart disease causes people to have hospital stays that last at least five days or more.[2]
- More than three million people have been victimized by and are living with the debilitating effects of a stroke.
- About five hundred thousand people have strokes each year.
- About one hundred fifty thousand people die of stroke each year.
- Hypertension is reported to affect sixty million Americans.
- Over five hundred million people have died in the last fifty years from preventable heart disease.
- Over four hundred thousand new cases of heart failure are diagnosed each year.
- Fifty thousand people die of heart failure each year.

The scientific and medical communities knew in 1941 that four out of five heart disease patients had low vitamin C levels, but chose to ignore it.[3] Prevention, reversal, and cure of heart disease are at hand now. But the medical community, pharmaceutical industry, government agencies, and health organizations want to continue to suppress and ignore this information. This small but frightening group of grim statistics only serves to affirm our belief that the conventional allopathic medical philosophy, the pharmaceutical industry, health educators, health associations, and organizations have failed miserably at their poorly advised and misguided attempts to reduce the incidence of, or cure, heart disease. Despite the fact that they have been given the knowledge, time and time again, they have failed miserably. What is their real interest?

Cardio Destruction: Debunking the "Cholesterol Is Killing Us" Myth

This is a truth we've been eager to share for a long time. The old, lame paradigm that cholesterol causes heart disease is laden with scientific error. We have evidence to show that this fundamental misunderstanding and biochemical naïveté of human biochemistry, as it relates to diet and nutrition, is incomplete and incorrect thinking. Remember our earlier discussion about cause and effect? Cholesterol does not cause heart disease. During the last two decades, the National Cholesterol Education Program, in conjunction with pharmaceutical companies and the medical community, has inaccurately brainwashed the public into believing that high cholesterol levels in the blood were the only serious major independent risk factor and predictor of heart disease. This gross miscarriage of information has been perpetuated at the expense of the lives of millions of people like you. Think of your family members and friends who could have been saved from this debilitating illness and premature death.

Often without warning, more than one million Americans, and more than twelve million people worldwide, unexpectedly become the victims of fatal heart attacks and strokes each year. Hundreds of thousands more are victims of strokes, heart attacks, blockages, and other forms of cardiovascular disease that cause severe damage and premature death. Untold thousands more escape death only to become prisoners of some disabling condition and/or impaired brain function. Typically undetectable until it's too late, cardiovascular disease develops silently and without warning. Whether we have high cholesterol and triglyceride levels or not, some experts encourage us to eat low-cholesterol, low-fat diets to reduce our risks, while other experts advise us to do practically the opposite. The fact is not everyone with high cholesterol has a heart attack or stroke. And many people with normal cholesterol levels do fall victim to cardiovascular disease. It's clear that other causes exist, causes more significant and imposing than high cholesterol levels alone. We know for certain that many factors collectively contribute to the onset and development of cardiovascular disease. Just when nearly everyone was convinced that cholesterol was the cause of heart disease, solid new scientific evidence points to the fact that cholesterol is a response and remedy to a cardiovascular injury, not its cause.

The most dangerous factors triggering cardiovascular accidents and disease are deficiencies of vitamin C, lysine, proline, and EFAs that initiate the deposition of lipoprotein(a) and cholesterol. Free radical damage caused by low antioxidant levels, nutritional deficiencies, arterial inflammation and stress, bacterial toxins and viruses, smoking, alcohol, and drugs also set the stage for *cardio destruction*. Many are considered major independent risk factors for heart disease, perhaps more significant than cholesterol. The good news is, these stealthlike, unrelenting biological terrorists can be controlled, reduced, or eliminated easily by nearly everyone. Don't be a victim!

How confusing all this information is! The French are healthier than we are even though they eat lots of fat and smoke lots of cigarettes. But they drink lots of red wine; eat more fresh fruit, vegetables, and garlic; and consume one-twentieth the amount of refined sugar than we do. The Japanese are much healthier than we are, too, although they eat a great deal of salty, pickled vegetables, soy sauces, and refined white rice. However, they consume large quantities of soy foods, fresh fish, green tea, and garlic, too. Their diet consists of much less refined sugar and saturated fat. Similar scenarios occur in other countries around the world.

Finally, a note about terminology: Throughout this book we will use the terms heart disease, cardiovascular disease, CVD, CAD, and other terms interchangeably to discuss diseases and conditions of the heart and/or cardiovascular system.

PART I

What Is Heart Disease and Why Do We Develop It?

THE HUMAN BODY IS DESIGNED TO TAKE PUNISHMENT. LOTS OF it. So much in fact that we can hardly think of anything else capable of withstanding the abuse that our bodies take in the course of a lifetime. Our cardiovascular system is the most resilient. It has a higher resistance to damage and takes much more punishment than any of our other organs, tissues, and structures. Although our arteries, capillaries, veins, and hearts are remarkably strong, pliant, and—most important—very, very forgiving, they can only withstand so much abuse. Our built-in repair mechanisms do their very best to maintain the integrity of the cardiovascular system. But there are limits. When the strain and pressure become too much to bear, the defects grow too large, the nutrient levels drop too low, the accidents and the injuries occur too frequently, then serious, sometimes irreversible, damage and destruction are inevitable.

Think about it. Isn't it really quite foolish and naive to believe that heart disease, America's number one killer, is caused by just one factor? And worse yet, to think that we base clinical evaluation of cardiovascular risk on the measurement of just one factor—cholesterol? Hardest of all to imagine and accept is the focus of the medical community. For over twenty years it has essentially done just that, turning cholesterol, your friend in time of need (and we always need cholesterol), into the unfortunate, misunderstood, and mistaken scapegoat for heart disease.

A person with high cholesterol levels has been treated like a prisoner on death row, but the prisoner has been falsely accused. Nearly all the focus and energy have been placed on measuring and controlling cholesterol levels, presuming that by lowering cholesterol the incidence of heart disease will decrease. Aiming at the bleachers when you want to throw the ball across home plate never really works. Focusing on cholesterol, an essential nutrient for many biochemical processes in the body, while ignoring the other factors that cause heart disease, will certainly continue to kill people by virtue of professional ignorance or neglect. This happens every day.

The complexity of the human body continually leads us to new discoveries about how it works. We should never forget that human biology and biochemistry are shaped by genetics, environment, food, and physical activity. These variables create a constantly changing pattern of metabolic activity that is slightly different for each person. They have created similar yet different metabolic and nutritional needs in each one of us. This brilliant concept was expounded and highlighted years ago by famed biochemist Roger Williams, Ph.D., who coined the term *bioindividuality*. In light of that, can just one entity—cholesterol— really be the "all-evil" cardiovascular villain?

The Cardiovascular System

YOUR HEART. VOLUMES HAVE BEEN WRITTEN ABOUT IT. IT IS THE symbol of life, love, and compassion, and the harbinger of impending death when it begins to fail or ceases to function. Far and away it is the most remarkable, fascinating, and complex organ in the human body. It's hard to imagine it is only a fist-sized muscle that sits near the center of your chest, silently beating without rest until . . . your "ticker" tape runs out!

In 1628, noted English physician William Harvey presented the first rudimentary description of our circulatory system. From then, we have come to learn that your heart is the silent master of your body and your life. Going mostly unnoticed, it beats, uninterrupted, on the average of sixty to eighty times per minute. In other words, about 100,000 times in twenty-four hours. It beats each day, 365 days a year, over thirty-six million times per year, for all the years of your life, never stopping until the end. For the average seventy-year-old it has pumped over two and one-half billion times! Remarkably, we hardly ever think about it except when we visit the doctor or personally experience a cardiovascular tragedy or witness one of someone we know.

Big Red

About the size of two clenched fists, the human heart is a hollow-chambered pump made of muscle called the myocardium that continuously pumps blood, circulating it throughout the body. It is stimulated to run by electrical currents and powered to feed about sixty thousand miles of arteries, capillaries, microcapillaries, and veins with blood that contains oxygen, nutrients, and hormones required for cellular respiration and energy. The farther away from the heart the vessels are located, the thinner they become. The most peripheral (outermost) microcapillaries are only one red blood cell thick. A single red blood cell in a microcapillary, now an inconceivable one-tenth the thickness of a human hair, has to compress and contort itself to fit and pass through. What abuse!

The heart is constructed of four chambers. The left and right atriums are the top two chambers and the left and right ventricles are the bottom two chambers. Then there is the aorta, the main artery carrying blood out of the heart, and the coronary arteries that supply blood to the heart. Two small areas of tissue called nodes—the sinus (sinoatrial) node and atrioventricular node—supply electrical impulses to fire the heart.

The sinus node, occupying a small area of the right atrium, is where each heartbeat begins. Here, much like a battery, an electrical force is discharged anywhere from sixty to one hundred times per minute. It is the "natural pacemaker" for the heart because it regulates the heartbeat. The electrically stimulated, rhythmic squeezing of the heart muscle (contractions) pumps blood out when the electrical impulse is discharged.

Blood returning from veins enters the right atrium and flows to the right ventricle where it is sent to the pulmonary artery to pick up oxygen from the lungs. Bright red blood, rich in oxygen taken on from the lungs, and nutrients absorbed through villi (little fingers in the small intestine) are pumped out of the heart into the aorta, the largest blood vessel in the cardiovascular system. The aorta feeds the carotid arteries, located on both sides of the neck, which nourish the brain with oxygen-rich blood. The abdominal aorta feeds the rest of body its supply of blood by circulating it throughout the body in arteries and smaller blood vessels known as capillaries.

Red blood cells in the blood deliver oxygen and nutrients to cells so that they can metabolize (burn) the nutrient fuel to create energy that the body can use. Once depleted of those nutrients and oxygen, dark red blood, filled with carbon dioxide and toxins given off as waste products of the energy-creating process, travels back to the heart through our venules and veins. And so the heart, via its circulatory plumbing system of arteries, arterioles, and capillaries, relentlessly delivers oxygen and nutrients to cells. The veins and venules remove harmful waste products of metabolism from the cells after energy has been produced.

The Pipeline: It's Your Plumbing, So Keep It Clean

At birth you were given clean, smooth arteries. Then genetics, diet, environment, and stress got in the way to clog your plumbing! Your arteries are constructed of three basic layers. The first layer is the *intima*. It is the innermost layer or lining over which the blood actually flows. This lining is also called the endothelium because it is composed of a single layer of protective endothelial cells. Molecules of glycosaminoglycans (GAGs), composed of 95 percent polysaccharides and 5 percent protein substances in connective tissue, form the extracellular medium that surrounds the cells. It is called the ground substance, the glue that holds cells together, acting as a first line of defense against injury and assisting with repair. Beneath the endothelium lies a support layer called the internal elastic membrane, made up of GAGs

5

and other gluelike compounds that support the endothelium, while separating it from smooth muscle cells in the media.

The second layer is the *media*. It is primarily composed of smooth muscle cells, with GAGs and ground substance molecules that provide support and elasticity.

The third layer is the *adventitia* or external elastic membrane. It is primarily made up of connective tissue called Type III collagen, one of five types of collagen found in the human body, and GAGs that also give elasticity and support.

The capillaries, some as thin as one red blood cell, are constructed solely of endothelial cells. This distinctive plumbing system pumps over 2,100 gallons of blood per day throughout the body and nourishes over three hundred trillion cells!

Blood: Your Magical "Life Juice"

This unique red liquid is the stuff that makes us nauseous when it comes out of our bodies unexpectedly, such as when we get a nasty nosebleed or cut. Like it or not, blood is the lifeline that transports vital biochemical substances to cells, tissues, organs and structures all over the body. Each of us has about 10½ pints of blood constantly flowing through their circulatory system. It is composed of three kinds of cells:

- Red blood cells (erythrocytes), about twenty-five trillion of them
- White blood cells (leukocytes), of different shapes and types, which defend against invading organisms
- Platelets, which are plate-shaped disks that trigger the blood-clotting mechanism to prevent loss of blood after injury

All three types of blood cells are suspended in plasma, a yellowish liquid that is 90 percent water and 10 percent glucose, salts, proteins, cholesterol, and other substances. Plasma's main job is to carry the three types of blood cells to their destinations.

Death: The Final Frontier

The inevitability of death and its occurrence as the culmination and finality of life are unchallenged. The ways in which it occurs and when within the human chronological life span it knocks on the door are factors that we, to a great extent, can control. We know that it is totally unnecessary for people to die, at the rate of two every minute of every day, from heart attacks, strokes, or other forms of cardiovascular disease when the knowledge, strategies, and techniques of proper cardiovascular care are at our fingertips. We can't stop the clock completely, but we can surely slow it down by maximizing the function and health of our hearts for a long and healthy lifetime.

We begin the journey by understanding the different types of heart disease and their real causes.

The Many Faces of Cardiovascular Disease (CVD)

I N 1912, JAMES B. HERRICK, M.D., FIRST DESCRIBED HEART disease as being caused by hardening of the arteries. Overall, cardiovascular disease is a group of conditions that interfere with the normal functioning of the heart and blood vessels.

Coronary Artery Disease (CAD)

By far, coronary artery disease is the most familiar type of cardiovascular disease and the most prevalent. Stiffening and hardening of the arteries is called arteriosclerosis. The accumulation of deposits (called plaques) on the artery walls is called atherosclerosis. Both are caused by the repeated cycle of:

- Injury (lesion) at a site on the artery wall
- Inflammation of the injured area
- Repair of the damage

The cycle begins with weak, thin, porous, inflexible, and inelastic artery walls coupled with endothelial dysfunction and weakness. This susceptibility of the endothelium (endothelial barrier cells between the blood and the first layer of the artery wall) initiates the damage. The endothelium, structurally weak from attack by physiological and biological cardioirritants, cannot resist the constant outward pressure of the blood at systole (when the heart pumps) and eventually ruptures or leaks. This injury is further aggravated by other cardioirritants and abnormalities.

Cardioirritants and Abnormalities

The most common cardioirritants and abnormalities are as follows:

- Unchecked free radicals
- Plaque accumulations on the artery wall infiltrated by low-density lipoprotein (LDL) cholesterol
- Oxidized LDL cholesterol
- Oxysterols (oxidized—biologically rusted—fats)
- Calcium
- Clots
- Improperly functioning valves
- Inflammation
- Poor electrical impulse transmissions
- Hypoxia (lack of oxygen)

These cardioirritants and abnormalities initiate the Cardiovascular Metabolic Repair Response—CMRR. Then, fatty streaks and deposits of lipoprotein(a), cholesterol, and oxidized cholesterol develop, often from childhood. This is the beginning of atherosclerosis, which causes the arteries, particularly the coronary arteries that supply oxygen and nutrients to the heart muscle, to become stiff and inelastic. The blood-filled inner orifice of the artery, called the lumen, continues to narrow as these fatty streaks slowly grow into atherosclerotic plaques that progressively block the flow of blood in the arteries. This hardening (arteriosclerosis) of the arteries and accumulation of fatty deposits on the artery walls (atherosclerosis) finally narrows the artery so much that blood flow stops. This can cause angina, heart attack (myocardial infarction—MI), or stroke. A plaque or a clot blocks the coronary artery; the rate of deposit varies by person.[1]

Anatomy of a Heart Attack: Are You Having the "Big One"?

In almost all cases, there are no advance warning signs of it. The last visit to the doctor was "good." Your cholesterol was a little high but nothing to worry about. You feel fine, just a little stressed out because, as usual, you are working a bit too hard. Then "it" happens, spontaneous as a lightning bolt from the sky. Your chest feels uneasily tight and there's lots of uncomfortable pressure on it, perhaps a squeezing feeling. And the pressure and pain stay for at least five to fifteen minutes, but usually more than one hour. The discomfort or pain may branch out into your neck, jaw, shoulders, or arms, particularly your left arm. You may or may not feel sweaty, nauseous, and lightheaded. Struggling to catch your breath is possible. Or, it may just seem like a terrible case of indigestion. You are the lucky one because you have symptoms. And those symptoms are a warning sign to get medical attention immediately. In 20 percent of MIs there are no symptoms at all. If this happens to you—seek immediate emergency treatment! Chances are you're having a heart attack!

What Happened?

When a heart attack occurs it means that vital heart muscle tissue has died or is dying as a result of oxygen starvation. Dramatically less oxygen is getting to the affected area of the heart. About 90 percent of the time this happens because one of the main coronary arteries surrounding the heart that supply it with oxygen and nutrients has been obstructed or closed by a blood clot, blocking the flow of blood. Or the artery has been narrowed by severe atherosclerosis, a 90 to 100 percent buildup of plaque that stops blood flow. In fewer cases, a severe spasm of the artery chokes off blood supply. As the heart muscle dies and the muscle membranes dissolve, they release an enzyme called CPK (creatine phosphokinase) and three other enzymes into the blood. CPK is immediately detectable and is a first biochemically diagnostic confirmation of a heart attack. Unattended heart attacks can easily result in unexpected, premature death.

They occur most often in middle-aged to elderly men and postmenopausal women. The chance of this happening is much more likely in those who have undiagnosed nutrient deficiencies, those who smoke, those who are obese, or those who have chronic high blood pressure or a family history of early heart disease. You know who you are! Start changing the odds now.

The Real Causes of CVD

With rare exception, all heart attacks are caused by atherosclerosis. According to the National Center for Health Statistics, over sixty-eight million Americans have some form of CVD. Many factors are constantly at work to negatively influence efficient cardiovascular function.[2] The first major study to identify cardiovascular risk factors was the Framingham Heart Study. It began in 1948, in Framingham, Massachusetts, and started with just 5,209 participants between thirty and

Culprits in the Development of Heart Disease	
Vitamin C deficiency	Elevated fibrinogen and
EFA deficiency	other clotting factors
Nutritional deficiencies	Arterial inflammation
Low antioxidant status	Adrenalin/cortisol
High circulating levels	High blood pressure
of free radicals	Diabetes
Lipoprotein(a)	Obesity
LDL cholesterol	Smoking
Triglycerides and other	Drugs
blood lipids (fats)	Alcohol
Blood sugar (glucose)	Stress
Insulin	Genetic defects
Homocysteine	

sixty-two years of age. The first director of the study, Dr. William Kannel, coined the term *cardiovascular risk factors*.

Cardiovascular Risk Factors: What Are They?

These are biochemical or physiological factors that contribute to the development of cardiovascular disease.

Cardiovascular Risk Markers There are biochemical or physiological factors that we can identify and measure to indicate the potential for, or presence of, cardiovascular disease. Many risk factors, such as lipoprotein(a) and cholesterol, are both risk factors and risk markers, because they contribute to, measure, and indicate the potential or presence of heart disease.

How this destruction takes place is illustrated in Figure 2.1.

Risk Markers

LDL cholesterol	Elevated fibrinogen and
Triglycerides	other clotting factors
Lipoprotein(a)	Glucose
Homocysteine	Insulin
CRP (C-reactive protein)	High blood pressure
Obesity	Diabetes

FIGURE 2.1 **Arteriosclerosis/Atherosclerosis/CVD**

The Chain of Events

Vitamin C deficiency + proline and lysine deficiency +
sulfur deficiency

Structurally deformed/damaged collagen or
insufficient collagen production

Weak, nonfibrous collagen matrix

Arterial instability + fragility + inflexibility =
endothelial dysfunction

Arterial injury (lesion) from	Insulin	Smoking
cardioirritating factors:	Adrenalin	Alcohol
Homocysteine	Viruses	Drugs
Glycation of glucose	Bacteria	Hypertension

Oxidative damage by free radicals

Arterial inflammation and elevated CRP (C-reactive protein)

Cardiovascular metabolic repair response (CMRR)

Deposition of lipoprotein(a) and cholesterol

Immune system response

Monocytes at injury/lesion sites become macrophages that collect
more lipoprotein(a)/cholesterol/lipids

A clotting response that sends platelets to the injury site, releasing
growth factors that stimulate smooth muscle cell migration from
media to intima and proliferation of smooth muscle cells in intima
that release cellular debris leading to deposition and accumulation
of more lipoprotein(a), oxidized LDL cholesterol, triglycerides,
fats, calcium

Growth of plaques

Rupture of artery—Blockage of artery in place—
Blockage by plaque break-off

Heart attack—Stroke—Angina—Hypertension—
Peripheral artery disease

The Development of Cardiovascular and Coronary Artery Disease

Now let's take a closer look at the steps we've shown in Figure 2.1. The innermost linings of the arteries, over which blood flows, are smooth at birth. But they are subject to a variety of ongoing assaults. They constantly take abusive pressure, especially each time the heart pumps blood out into the circulatory system. And thousands of different biomolecules, nutrients, and foreign substances continuously go whizzing by.

In a fantasy cardiovascular world, the artery linings would be like Teflon, impervious to practically everything. Blood and all that flows through it would never do any damage at all. But the lining is not Teflon, or the hardest steel. Instead, it is living, breathing, soft, flexible tissue that is highly susceptible and vulnerable to all sorts of attacks. However, the degree to which it is susceptible is the prime consideration.

When ample vitamin C, lysine, proline, sulfur, copper, and vitamin B_6 are present, we make enough good quality collagen to produce a strong, dense, heavily cross-linked collagen matrix (network) that is usually impervious to the physical and chemical stresses that would otherwise cause it to rupture and become damaged. Only a slight arterial abrasion would result from normal wear and tear of blood constantly rushing by.

Unfortunately, because human beings lost their ability to manufacture vitamin C internally during prehistoric times, we are constantly undersupplied with it. Therefore, we harbor a lifelong chronic vitamin C deficiency (hypoascorbemia). We cannot produce it on demand when we need to make more collagen, neutralize free radicals, or support aggressive immune function. As our requirement for vitamin C increases in response to factors entering the blood from food, air, and water, our meager supply becomes quickly drained. Very little, if any, vitamin C remains in our blood—a bad situation turned worse. The small amounts available in a typical American diet are nowhere near enough to do all the metabolic work.

Our arteries are now very vulnerable to damage. We try to make collagen, but there is not enough vitamin C to do it properly. A small amount of collagen is made, but it is deformed, weak, and damaged. Without vitamin C and other antioxidants, free radicals build their armies rapidly. The artery walls are in serious trouble. First, free radicals and all those zooming things destroy the endothelial cell lining on the artery wall.

Endothelial Dysfunction: The Walls Start Tumbling

Endothelial dysfunction is a technical term used to describe the inability of the endothelium to maintain structural integrity of the intima of the artery. The endothelium is the lining of special cells, called endothelial barrier cells, that lie between blood and the first layer of the artery wall called the intima. The first major function of these cells is to protect the intima from cardioirritants and injury. The second major function of the endothelium is to control blood pressure.

Endothelial dysfunction is marked by a lack of flexibility in the blood vessels and a failure to dilate (expand) under pressure when necessary. Normal dilation occurs by the production of nitric oxide and a prostaglandin called prostacyclin, a powerful vasodilator and the most potent inhibitor of platelet aggregation. Atherosclerosis and hyperlipidemia (excess blood lipids) impair endothelial function, as does Syndrome X (see pages 103–104) and diets high in saturated fats. An overproduction of endothelin (a vasoconstrictor) is also responsible for endothelial dysfunction and is a major cause of high blood pressure.

Information from Anesthesia Clinics of North America reveals that overproduction occurs when endothelial cells produce endothelium derived relaxing factor (EDRF), more commonly known as nitric oxide. What is the importance of this? Nitric oxide is the primary endogenous (internally produced) vasodilator for the arteries. Simply, nitric oxide is produced within the cells and acts to relax and dilate the arteries, which lowers the resistance of flowing blood. Less resistance equals less pressure, thus lower blood pressure. Nitric oxide production diminishes with age, the onset of diabetes, high cholesterol, smoking, and inactivity. Inhibition of or inability to produce nitric oxide causes hypertension (high blood pressure).[3] In a recent study, researchers discovered that supplementation with folic acid protected healthy subjects from endothelial damage caused by dietary fat and simultaneously decreased the production of free radicals. The lesson here appears to be that increased intake of folic acid can protect us from high blood pressure and vascular damage and disease.[4]

One major study conducted in 1999 by S. Schroeder, reported in the *American Heart Journal*, revealed that a positive determination of endothelial dysfunction was a sensitive and specific screening test to predict the presence of coronary artery disease. The test used noninvasive ultrasound diagnostics to determine something researchers call FMD (flow-mediated dilation), which essentially tells how much the artery dilates under the changing pressure of blood flow. Endothelial dysfunction was defined as the inability of the artery to dilate more than 4½ percent from normal.[5]

Now back to those zooming things we mentioned above. They find defects in the collagen and vigorously attack them. Other biomolecules attack, too. Homocysteine, glucose, insulin, adrenalin, bacteria, viruses, and chemicals in smoke, drugs, and alcohol join in the attack. The pressure of emerging blood presses intensely against the weakened artery walls. They can't resist it and become unstable, fragile, and inflexible. Deficiencies of EFAs, needed to keep cell membranes soft, contribute to the rigidity. Cracks begin to appear. Injured areas become inflamed and C-reactive protein, a biomarker of that inflammation, becomes elevated. If the body does not repair the injury, hemorrhaging occurs. When this happens along carotid arteries of the neck or arteries and capillaries in the brain, the hemorrhaging is known as a stroke. Unstopped, death is likely. On the other hand, the body initiates what we call the Cardiovascular Metabolic Repair Response (CMRR).

Cardiovascular Metabolic Repair Response

The Cardiovascular Metabolic Repair Response (CMRR) is a two-pronged defense. On the one side, your liver begins to send its genetic repair "patch and plug" molecules, lipoprotein(a), to the injury site. It also dispatches "Mr. Fix-it," LDL cholesterol, there. And the very dangerous oxidized LDL cholesterol makes its way to the injury site, too. These three lipoproteins literally fill in the damaged areas, much the same way as you would plaster a crack or hole in your wall. Once this patch is established, it becomes a magnet for more lipoprotein(a) and more cholesterol. It also attracts other fats, such as triglycerides, and calcium circulating in the blood to the site. These deposited lipoproteins are not very fluid and stiffen the artery wall. With calcium as a component, the deposits, first meant to repair and prevent uncontrolled rupture and bleeding, become the Dr. Jekyll and Mr. Hyde of the artery wall. They now continue to attract artery-stiffening substances. Meanwhile, the immune response is set into motion at the first signs of plaque buildup.

In healthy tissue, repeated injuries to endothelial cells cause the formation of sticky cell adhesion molecules (CAMs). These CAMs initiate a healing and repair process by placing a biochemical ID tag on the cell. They identify the enemy and send a signal for help. White blood cells (monocytes) are summoned to the injury site and attach to the blood vessel lining by squeezing among the endothelial cells. This causes inflammation in the tissue below. The monocytes change themselves into macrophages, the "garbage collector" white blood cells of the immune system. Hungry macrophages and CAMs begin to soak up cholesterol and other fats. CAMs collect more LDL cholesterol, lipoprotein(a), and platelets that travel to the injury site to do their repairs. A fibrous cap (protein coating) forms over the developing plaque. Macrophages also release growth factors that stimulate the movement of smooth muscle cells from the middle layer of the artery to the innermost layer, the one that has just been damaged. The smooth muscle cells multiply on the intima, causing them to drop debris that contributes to plaque formation. Simultaneously, the clotting cells (platelets) also move to the injury site to form a clot and repair the damage. Eventually, the macrophages collect so much cholesterol and fats that they develop a foamy appearance and are logically called foam cells. Finally, they burst and their contents spill out into the plaque, already filled with cholesterol, oxidized cholesterol, lipoprotein(a), platelets, and smooth muscle cell debris.

What a mess! One of two things can happen next. The plaque can grow in place, building up and progressively occupying more space in the opening of the artery. Blood flow diminishes. This eventually causes intermittent interruptions in blood flow called ministrokes, or transient ischemic attacks (TIAs), and angina. Or the plaque will finally block the artery, completely choking off blood supply to the heart. That's a heart attack!

Blockages that are stationary can be detected with diagnostics such as an echocardiogram, CAT scan, Ultrafast CT scan, or angiogram. The other scenario is far worse. Younger developing plaques that are not hard or large cannot usually be detected diagnostically because they flex with the pressure of blood. They pose a far greater danger because we don't know they are there and they can break away at any time. Developing plaques can travel to the carotid arteries or brain and the clot (thrombus) can block blood flow to brain cells, causing a stroke. If the plaques block a coronary artery, a heart attack will occur. It's not a pretty scenario, but it does happen without warning every day to thousands of people.

This can be easily prevented! Sufficient vitamin C, lysine, proline, sulfur, copper, and vitamin B_6 will build and maintain superstrong arteries. An ample supply of EFAs will keep the cell membranes soft, pliable, flexible, elastic, and ready to withstand the constant intense pressure of blood. Sufficient antioxidants will prevent relentless attacks by cardiodestructive free radicals. B vitamins will prevent excesses of homocysteine.

Angina

This is the miserable, recurring, and mild to excruciating chest pain that millions of Americans experience every day. Typically, there is a squeezing pain or the sensation of pressure and heaviness due to an insufficient supply of oxygen (hypoxia) being transported to the heart muscle. The pain, usually lasting anywhere from one to twenty minutes, may radiate into the left arm or shoulder. The atherosclerosis of hard, plaque-covered arteries is almost always the villain that causes it by decreasing the opening in the artery through which blood can flow. Less blood flow means less oxygen, and that lack of oxygen causes chest pain. Angina can be reduced with dietary measures and natural therapies. Recent findings from the National Health and Nutrition Examination Survey III revealed that carotenoid supplements, such as beta-carotene, alpha-carotene and beta-cryptoxanthin, were associated with about a 50 percent reduction of the risk for angina pectoris.

High Blood Pressure and Tight Arteries: Are You Ready to Burst?

Hypertension causes no symptoms and is the silent killer reported to affect an incredible sixty million Americans! Over half of them (54.3 percent) are aged sixty-five to seventy four.[6] When blood vessels are narrowed, the heart must work harder to pump and push the blood through them. High blood pressure is a causative factor in forcing blood fats and cholesterol into the artery wall. Over time, increased blood pressure can cause a ballooning of the artery wall (aneurysm). Eventually, high blood pressure will scar small arteries (arterioles), reducing the availability of oxygen- and nutrient-rich blood to specific body areas.

High blood pressure is caused by a variety of factors. The heart pumps blood into the aorta, causing intense pressure against artery walls. This is called systolic pressure (the high number). The pressure of blood against artery walls when the heart rests is called diastolic pressure (the low number). Most physicians seem to be concerned primarily with the low number, but both are just as important. In fact, Dr. W. B. Kannel of Boston University School of Medicine reviewed the contributions of both systolic and diastolic blood pressure to the risk of cardiovascular disease. By examining the evidence available from the Framingham Heart Study and the change in attitudes toward systolic pressure while conducting the study, Dr. Kannel's review points out that in the past, systolic pressure was considered an innocent accompaniment to arterial stiffening. However, epidemiologic data illustrated that systolic pressure is in fact more important than diastolic pressure in determining cardiovascular events. Dr. Kannel goes on to say that a mild elevation of systolic blood pressure, even without increased diastolic pressure, poses an increased risk of CVD. The risk increases further if glucose intolerance, dyslipidemia (blood fat imbalances), insulin resistance, cardiac hypertrophy (shrinking heart muscle), or obesity are present. Finally, Dr. Kannel warns that reliance on diastolic pressure alone is misleading, as systolic pressure is a powerful predictor of cardiovascular disease along with other risk factors.[7]

What Causes High Blood Pressure?

There are many causes of high blood pressure, but among the most common are the following:

Endothelial Dysfunction Endothelial dysfunction is the inability of your arteries to expand against the pressure of blood being pumped and pushed out from the heart; this causes tremendous resistance. This resistance is the blood pressure.

EFA Deficiency A lack of essential fatty acids in the cell membranes of arterial and capillary cells renders them stiff and inflexible. This rigidity creates significantly more resistance to the flow and pressure of blood emerging from the heart and increases the pressure it exerts. Cell membranes that are deficient in EFAs also restrict the entry of nutrients, oxygen, and other fatty acids that are needed to provide energy and prevent the elimination of metabolic wastes, toxins, and carbon dioxide.

High Sodium to Potassium Ratio in the Blood Perhaps the biggest culprits and the easiest imbalances to correct are the amounts of potassium and sodium in the blood.

Lowering sodium intake alone will only help minimally. Additional dietary potassium is needed. But the typical ratio of potassium to sodium in the American diet is less than 1:2. We are consuming twice as much sodium (salt) as potassium! The consensus of research concludes that to maintain health a 5:1 ratio of potassium to sodium is needed. We believe, as do many natural health experts, that an even higher ratio is optimal, especially for heart health. If you consume a diet rich in fruits, vegetables, legumes, and grains, your potassium/sodium ratio can be as high 100:1, since most fruits and vegetables have a natural potassium/sodium ratio of 50:1 or more.

The Committee on Recommended Dietary Allowances tells us that it is safe to consume 1.9 to 5.6 grams of potassium per day. This is 1,900 to 5,600 milligrams per day, primarily from dietary sources. Potassium is the most important electrolyte (a mineral salt that conducts electricity when dissolved in water) in our body fluids. It maintains blood pressure; heart, kidney and adrenal function; muscle and nerve cell function; and water balance and distribution, while preserving acid/base balance.

Ninety-five percent of potassium does its work inside the cells, while sodium is present outside the cells in fluids and blood. The cells pump sodium out and pump potassium in. Dozens of studies show that low potassium–high sodium diets are major causes of heart disease and cancer. Conversely, high potassium–low sodium diets are cardio and cancer protective.[8] Caffeinated coffee, alcohol intake, lack of exercise, stress, smoking, obesity, high-sugar diets, and diets high in saturated fat with low EFA intake are additional culprits in the elevation of blood pressure.

Diet, natural remedies, exercise, and stress reduction techniques are more effective than prescription drugs for high blood pressure, many of which cause the very thing they are attempting to prevent— a heart attack. While prescription medications for high blood pressure are being provided in record-breaking numbers, the Multiple Risk Factor Intervention Trial (MRFIT) has clearly proven that prescription medications do not offer any benefit to those who have borderline to moderate hypertension.

Stroke

Stroke is known as ischemic heart disease and cerebrovascular accident (CVA). The three major forms of stroke are: thrombotic, hemorrhagic, and embolitic. Transient Ischemic Attacks (TIAs), also called ministrokes, affect more than two and one-half million Americans.

In advanced cardiovascular disease, atherosclerotic buildup causes blockage in carotid arteries supplying blood to the brain, literally choking off the blood supply. A thrombotic stroke occurs when a clot (thrombus) forms in a carotid artery and blocks blood flow, cutting off oxygen and nutrients. Approximately 80 percent of strokes are this type. The other 18 percent are hemorrhagic strokes that occur when

---

What Is Heart-Healthy Blood Pressure?

Normal: 120 (Systolic) over 80 (Diastolic)
Borderline High: 120–160 over 90–94
Mild High: 140–160 over 95–104
Moderate high: 140–180 over 105–114
Severe high: 160+ over 115+

If your blood pressure is regularly borderline high or above, begin the program for a healthy heart contained in Part IV and consult your physician or health care provider.

---

the artery leaks or bursts, interrupting blood flow to the brain. Least common is the embolic stroke, which takes place when a clot formed in an arteries or the heart travels and lodges in an artery of the brain. TIAs are temporary interruptions of blood flow to the brain lasting typically only a few minutes to an hour. They do, however, cause temporary neurological damage. This interruption resolves itself and does not cause any permanent damage, but it is not by any means to be ignored. Immediate medical attention should be sought, as TIAs are excellent predictors of future TIAs and the strong possibility of a full-blown stroke.

One of the contributing factors to a stroke is carotid artery stenosis, a narrowing of the carotid arteries that provide blood to the brain. Homocysteine was found to increase the risk of this narrowing and consequently the risk of stroke. Jacob Selhub, Ph.D., of the U.S. Department of Agriculture, Human Nutrition Research Center on Aging at Tufts University, Boston, conducted a study of 1,041 seniors. He discovered that low concentrations of vitamin B_6, vitamin B_{12}, and folic acid, along with high blood concentrations of homocysteine, are associated with a higher risk of carotid artery stenosis in the elderly. He further concluded that this significantly increases the risk of stroke.

Ten Tips for Lowering Your Blood Pressure Now

1. Trim the fat—attain ideal body weight. Excess body weight forces the heart to pump harder and faster than intended. This intensified pumping means higher pressure exerted against artery walls.

2. Increase the potassium to sodium ratio in your diet: Increase the quantity of plant foods in your diet while reducing the quantity of animal foods. This will shift the ratio from sodium-rich to potassium-rich foods and lower your pressure.

3. Take EFA supplements and eat EFA–rich foods. Omega-3 EFAs (flax oil/seeds, walnuts, fish oils, fatty fish), omega-6 EFAs (nut, seed, vegetable oils), and garlic are plentiful sources.

4. Eat more vegetables and less meat. Plant-based diets are naturally rich in potassium while low in sodium. Studies show that vegetarians typically have a lower blood pressure and lower risk of heart disease than nonvegetarians.[9]

5. Try a salt replacement alternative that uses potassium chloride instead of sodium chloride.

6. Take extra magnesium. In 1983, at the Department of Internal Medicine, University Hospital, Ume University, Sweden, systolic and diastolic pressures decreased significantly in patients that were hypertensive or had congestive heart failure when they received magnesium supplementation.[10] This hypotensive (blood pressure–lowering) effect, reported in the *American Journal of Hypertension*, was repeated in a seventeen-patient study in 1993 by Wester and L. Widman. They noted that as magnesium supplementation increased, systolic pressure decreased and blood vessel tone normalized. This was attributed to magnesium's action as a natural calcium

channel blocker, preventing the constriction of blood vessels.[11]

7. Get regular exercise. Exercise increases the efficiency and pumping capacity of the heart. That means less pressure against artery walls, less often.

8. Stop smoking now! Few words are necessary here. Smoking raises blood pressure, poisons the blood, and overloads the liver.

9. Reduce stress. Stress will surely raise your blood pressure. As your level of tension, anxiety, anger, or fear increases, so does the production of stress hormones like adrenalin and cortisol. Your heart rate increases and your heart beats more powerfully than normal. This increases pressure on the artery walls. Relax!

10. Check your blood pressure often. We strongly urge you to monitor your blood pressure regularly. Since blood pressure changes constantly, actually every few seconds, one reading in the doctor's office while you are stressed and anxious is not a good indicator of your accurate average blood pressure. It is better to measure it regularly at home and take an average of the readings. If your blood pressure is consistently high, consult your doctor.

Finally, it was shown that vitamin supplementation including vitamin B_{12}, vitamin B_6, and folic acid brought the elevated homocysteine levels back down into the normal range.[12]

One of the major factors affecting stroke risk is diet, particularly the quantity of fruits and vegetables consumed. The 1995 study by Matthew W. Gillman, M.D, at the Department of Ambulatory Care and Prevention, Harvard Medical School, Boston, Massachusetts, observed that there was an inverse association between the development of stroke in men aged forty-five to sixty-five and their consumption of fruits and vegetables. The risk of stroke decreased by 22 percent for each additional three servings of fruit and vegetables consumed per day. He attributed that result to the antioxidant effect and its ability to reduce oxidation of LDL cholesterol and consequently the amount of LDL available to be taken up by arterial lesions.[13]

Heart Failure

It's a slow process. In this type of heart disease, the heart becomes stiff and fatigued from overwork. Heart muscle strength is diminished due to repeated injuries, lesion formation, and damage from heart attacks. Often, there is too much resistance caused by stiff, inelastic arteries clogged with atherosclerotic plaque buildup. Long-term chronic hypertension; narrowed exit valves, especially in the aorta, along with other leaky valves; viral infections; and alcohol-induced damage are the contributing factors. Eventually, the heart has very little power to pump blood and does so with insufficient force, finally leading to a complete halt.

Arrhythmias

Arrhythmias are a group of irregular heartbeat patterns of different types, including missed beats, skipped beats, extra beats, atrial fibrillation, ventricular fibrillation, tachychardia, bradychardia, and others. The heart's battery power, responsible for correct beating rhythm, is controlled by the sinus (SA) and atrioventricular (AV) nodes. Arrhythmias occur when the electrical system in the heart goes out of sync—literally haywire.

Valvular Heart Disease

This develops when one, several, or all of the valves in the heart malfunction because of stenosis (narrowing) or prolapse (improper closing). It occurs most times on the left side of heart, from stenosis, prolapse, or regurgitation (incomplete closing) of the valves. Valvular heart disease ultimately leads to heart failure. The most common form of valvular heart disease is peripheral vascular disease (PVD), which diminishes the supply of blood to the arms and legs. Advanced PVD is painful and impedes the ability to walk. Smoking is the biggest risk factor for PVD and one that can easily be controlled.

Cardiomyopathy:
Heart Muscle Diseases

Cardiomyopathy is the name of a group of primary diseases of the heart in which there is thickening of the heart muscle and the replacement of good heart muscle with rigid muscle that prevents proper function. Cardiomyopathy in childhood, often caused by energy-production defects in the energy-producing mitochondria of heart cells, is a cause of many deaths in children. Carnitine is needed to transport fats into the mitochondria where they are burned for energy. Given in supplemental form, l-carnitine, a natural substance essential for mitochondrial energy production, can improve or resolve childhood cardiomyopathy.[14]

Inflammatory Heart Diseases

There are three primary types of inflammatory heart disease:

Pericarditis: This is an inflammation of the outer membrane of the heart caused by a virus or infection.

Myocarditis: This occurs when the heart muscle becomes inflamed for unknown causes, perhaps secondary to a viral condition.

Endocarditis: This is an inflammation of the inner lining of the heart or valve caused by a bacterial infection.

Congenital Defects

From the eighth to tenth weeks after conception, the fetal heart fully develops. By the time it is no bigger than a peanut, any congenital defects destined to surface at birth are already present. Valve damage and holes in muscular tissue separating chambers are the most common congenital defects. A pinched aorta, a narrowed aorta, or "blue baby" syndrome (when part of the blood that is returning from the body does not pick up oxygen in the lungs because the aorta and pulmonary artery are reversed) are others. Each year, about twenty-five thousand babies are born with these defects and about 5,500 infant deaths occur each year as a result.

What You Should Know About Aspirin, Heart Disease, and Heart Attacks

Many doctors now prescribe low doses of aspirin to prevent first and second heart attacks. Why? Simply put, aspirin has been shown to produce antiplatelet activity—a biological chain of events that inhibits the production of localized hormonelike substances (prostaglandins such as thromboxane) that initiate a blood-clotting cascade. Aspirin's antiplatelet (anticlotting) activity prevents platelets from forming clots that can clog arteries. It's the remedy that practically every doctor recommends these days for primary prevention of a heart attack if you've never had one and secondary prevention if you already have.

Aspirin. It's a Good Idea, Right? Well, Maybe Not

Aspirin is without a doubt easy to take, inexpensive, and readily available without a prescription. But it only addresses one singular aspect of your cardiovascular risk, which is the possibility of platelet aggregation to form blood clots. The medical and pharmaceutical gurus out there making millions of bucks forgot all the other factors. Aspirin is a well-known and documented gastric irritant that can easily upset the stomach lining and cause bleeding in many people. This is especially true for those known to have, or suspect a family history of, gastric problems such as stomach ulcers. Aspirin is also an allergic substance for many people who have salicylate allergies. Finally, aspirin thins the blood and is not advised for those who have had a stroke or TIAs, or who have a family history of hemorrhagic stroke.

And Does It Really Work?

The standard recommendation for prevention, a baby aspirin (81 mg) per day or every other day, is not so sure to help. According to world-recognized naturopathic physician Michael Murray, M.D., coauthor of the *Encyclopedia of Natural Medicine*, nearly fifteen thousand people in seven studies who suffered a heart attack were monitored for the use of aspirin to prevent a second one. Not one study demonstrated a significant reduction in mortality.[15] Go natural! Dr. Murray tells us that the Lifestyle Heart Study conducted by Dean Ornish, M.D., indicated that diet was more effective than aspirin for preventing the recurrence of heart attacks.

Meanwhile, Grapes Prevent Heart Attacks!

Numerous studies prove conclusively that resveratrol, the potent antioxidant polyphenol found in red wine, exerts extremely aggressive, powerful antiplatelet activity. This suggests a lesser chance of blood clotting and incidence of heart attack or stroke. And it likely explains why the French have a lower rate of heart disease and heart attacks than other cultures.[16] Some unconfirmed research suggests that ethanol, the alcohol in wine, might have some very mild antiplatelet activity. But the dangers of alcohol for the liver far outweigh this one possible benefit, although occasional moderate wine consumption is not generally harmful to most healthy people.

Do You Need Bypass?

Should you plug the leak and forget the plumbing? By now you understand that the cardiovascular system is a complex pump and plumbing system that can't afford breakdowns, downtime, and leaks. If the whole system has a nasty, clogging buildup, what good is repairing or replacing just a few small sections? Yet the medical community is quick to recommend bypass surgery as a way of repairing clogged arteries. Diagnostic and surgical statistics show that many of these bypass surgeries are not necessary and carry with them a great degree of risk for failure, additional damage, or death. Just say no to bypass surgery unless urgently necessary.

Bypass Surgery and Coronary Angioplasty: Lifesavers?

Here's the scenario. First, the cardiologist examines the patient and immediately bypasses dietary changes, supplements, chelation therapy, exercise recommendations, and stress reduction techniques as first lines of noninvasive defense. He opts instead to go directly for your wallet and your emotions by telling you the other methods won't work in your serious situation. He then recommends bypass surgery as the answer to your problems, smoothly bypassing the severity of the risks. He'd rather perform an expensive and life-threatening repair job than really eliminate the cause of the problem.

Bypass him. Get another opinion from a cardiologist who integrates natural approaches.

Why Traditional Medical Thinking and Surgery Don't Work

The intent of bypass surgery is to bypass one or more coronary arteries that have become severely clogged with plaque to the point that blood flow is very restricted or completely blocked. Usually, veins from the leg are removed and implanted around the heart. After removing the blocked section of artery, one end of the implanted vein is attached to the aorta and the other end attached back to the coronary artery. This bypasses the blockage, ensuring uninterrupted blood flow.

Bypass surgery does not fully solve the problem. It is a localized repair technique that has a 50 percent failure rate. In many cases the new bypass vessel forms a clot and blocks blood flow again. Restenosis (re-closing and blockage of the repaired artery) occurs. The new bypass vessel develops plaque and becomes blocked. The arteries close again! Restenosis initiates the deposition of lipoprotein(a) all over again, and lipoprotein(a) is the greatest factor causing restenosis.[17] The rate of restenosis after bypass surgery is 15 to 30 percent within the first year. The risk of heart attack while on the operating table for bypass surgery is 5 percent of patients and 40 percent of high-risk patients.[18] Two percent of bypass surgery patients suffer irreversible neurological damage, paralysis, loss of speech, and blindness. Psychological trauma is common. Angiography, a primary test to determine the location and severity of a blockage, is itself dangerous.

Coronary Angioplasty

In contrast to bypass, coronary angioplasty is a procedure that actually squeezes the plaques flat against the artery wall (balloon angioplasty) or scrapes them away. These procedures are not safe either because they cause mechanical damage inside the artery, resulting in regrowth of deposits in the same place as before, or the formation of a clot. And as we mentioned earlier, younger developing plaques are susceptible to rupture at anytime, even during the procedure.

Chelation Therapy: A Better Way

Intravenous (IV) chelation therapy is a nonsurgical treatment that improves circulatory and metabolic function. It removes toxic metals, such as lead and cadmium, and abnormally located copper and iron deposits. Contrary to popular belief, IV chelation therapy does not remove calcium that is lodged in plaques, but it will remove calcium circulating in the blood. This effectively limits the calcium that can actually attach to plaques.

The therapy is performed by giving an IV solution of EDTA (ethylene-diamine-tetra-acetic acid), a synthetic amino acid, over a three- to four-hour period, once per week for ten to twenty weeks. Chelation, from the Greek for "claw," uses the injected solution to grab loosely bound and free-floating metal ions, removing them from the bloodstream and artery walls.

- Chelation, by binding to toxic metals, reduces the production of free radicals.
- Chelation increases blood flow, improves cholesterol ratios, and lowers blood fats.
- Chelation lowers blood pressure.
- Chelation reduces unhealthy cross-linkages of metal ions to proteins, thereby relaxing vessels and increasing blood flow.
- Chelation reduces circulating calcium, slowing its deposition in artery walls.
- EDTA restores the production of prostacyclin, a hormone that prevents spasms of the heart and arteries, while reducing platelet stickiness.
- EDTA reduces the rate of free radical reactions, by removing metals that oxidize fats.
- EDTA reduces free radical activity by a millionfold, according to Elmer Cranton, M.D., author of *Bypassing Bypass*.[19]

THREE

Women and Heart Disease

YOU HARDLY EVER HEAR OF A YOUNG WOMAN HAVING A HEART attack or stroke before menopause. And most people also have the mistaken notion that heart disease and heart attacks are a "guy" thing. That's because women typically have heart attacks, on average, ten years later than men. Women appear to be almost fully protected from cardiovascular risk before menopause, magically escaping by reason of their femininity. Although there are many similarities between women and men when it comes to heart disease, differences do exist.

Estrogen's Protective Effect

Fact is, a high level of estrogen, present in most premenopausal women, is the reason they are protected from cardiovascular disease. Women taking hormone replacement therapy (HRT) seem to have similar protection. A 1998 study conducted in the Department of Nutrition at Brigham and Women's Hospital, Boston, found that estrogen lowered lipoprotein(a) in the blood. The study, while admitting that the mechanism by which estrogen lowers lipoprotein(a) in the blood is not well understood, suggests that the reduced ability of lipoprotein(a) to enter into blood plasma could contribute to lower CVD rates in women taking estrogen.

Another study by Su and Campos is significant because it clearly pointed out that markers of inflammation are important predictors of cardiovascular risk in women. Previous studies were conducted only on middle-aged men.[1] High triglyceride levels in women correlate to heart attacks more often than in men. Between the ages of forty-five and sixty-four, one woman in nine develops some form of CVD. Women who have heart attacks are twice as likely to die as men. Studies show that within the first year after a heart attack, 31 percent of men died and 39 percent of women died!

Women are more affected by and at more risk from two factors, smoking and diabetes. Smoking reduces levels of cardioprotective estrogen and HDL cholesterol in the blood. A woman who smokes and uses oral contraceptives is forty times more likely to have a heart attack than those who use neither. Diabetes, which is more prevalent in women than in men, results in women having lower levels of HDL (high-density lipoprotein) cholesterol, which reduces their ability to remove dangerous excess LDL cholesterol from the blood. HDL cholesterol in the blood scoops up and removes the excess LDL cholesterol that causes atherosclerotic buildups.

It is believed that estrogen protects premenopausal women by increasing their levels of HDL. In premenopausal women, HDL cholesterol levels are remarkably higher than in men of the same age. Estrogen also prevents arteries from constricting and causing high blood pressure. During and after menopause, as estrogen levels decline, the protective effect diminishes with it. Postmenopausal women who take estrogen reduce their risk of heart attack by 33 to 50 percent.[2]

Mild obesity in women dramatically increases the chances of a heart attack. In one study of women who were 30 percent above ideal weight, obesity caused 70 percent of the heart attacks.

Antioxidants have a strong cardioprotective effect on women, too. A study conducted in the early 1990s by noted researcher Meir Stampfer, at the Channing Laboratory and the Division of Preventive Medicine at Harvard Medical School, monitored over 87,000 female nurses between the ages of thirty-four and fifty-nine who were free of diagnosed cardiovascular disease. One of Stampfer's conclusions was that for those women who took vitamin E in supplement form, the risk of developing coronary artery disease was approximately 40 percent lower than for women who did not supplement. In addition to that, women who took the vitamin E supplements demonstrated a significant increase in the ability of LDL cholesterol to resist oxidation, as opposed to no increase in resistance for those who did not supplement. Stampfer's findings show that increased amounts of vitamin E, beyond levels obtainable in the diet, appear necessary to prevent oxidation of LDL cholesterol.[3]

The natural onset of menopause increases heart attack risk. When menopause is induced by removal of the ovaries, the risk rises significantly.

Pregnancy-Induced Heart Disease

Pregnancy increases blood volume by about 40 percent, placing an extra workload on the heart. For normal, healthy women, the stresses and strains on the heart are in many ways like a strenuous exercise workout.

But hormonal and circulatory changes during pregnancy can induce hypertension. This usually occurs in the last trimester and fades quickly after delivery. If there is persistent hypertension with edema (swelling) in the legs, or protein in the urine, a condition called pre-eclampsia occurs. Without medical attention, it can develop into eclampsia, causing convulsions and seizures.[4]

FOUR

Blood Chemistry, Screening, and Diagnostic Tests

THE TESTS LISTED BELOW ARE DESIGNED TO MONITOR YOUR risks and progress. Blood tests and screening tests are available in the doctor's office, clinic, or hospital. The doctor in the office, clinic, or hospital performs blood pressure, heart rate, and carotid artery palpation tests, and draws blood for lab analysis. Electrocardiograms, exercise stress tests, and echocardiograms are offered in some offices and clinics and are always performed in the hospital. The Ultrafast CT scan is offered in select hospitals.

These tests tell us if specific markers of cardiovascular health and disease are within normal range.

Screening for Lipids

HDL cholesterol

LDL cholesterol

VLDL (very low density lipoprotein) cholesterol

Triglycerides

Lipoprotein(a)

Tests for Other Factors

C-reactive protein

Fibrinogen

Clotting/prothrombin time

Potassium

Glucose

HbA1c—Glycohemoglobin

Sodium

Magnesium

Ferritin

Screening and Diagnostic Tests

Blood pressure

Heart rate

Carotid artery palpation

Pulse oximetry

Exercise stress test

Electrocardiogram (EKG)

Echocardiogram

Ultrafast CT scan

The Tests

Lipoprotein(a)

This blood test measures circulating blood levels of lipoprotein(a), the adhesive form of LDL cholesterol.

- 0 to 20 mg/dl suggests a low risk of cardiovascular disease. Dietary and lifestyle changes, along with appropriate supplementation, are advised while risk is still low.
- 20 to 40 mg/dl suggests a moderate/medium risk of cardiovascular disease. Dietary and lifestyle changes, along with appropriate supplementation, are strongly urged while risk is present but moderate.
- 40+ mg/dl suggests a high risk of cardiovascular disease. Dietary and lifestyle changes, along with appropriate supplementation and diagnostic monitoring by a physician, are immediately advised to rapidly reduce the risk of emerging serious cardiovascular disease or cardiovascular accident.

Homocysteine

This test measures circulating blood levels of homocysteine, the nonessential amino acid. Current bionutritional research suggests that:

- 6 micromoles per liter of homocysteine in the blood represent low to no risk of cardiovascular disease.
- 10 micromoles per liter indicate an increased risk.
- 13 micromoles per liter are considered very dangerous.
- 13+ micromoles per liter warn that heart attack or stroke is just waiting to happen.

Sufficient supplementation with folic acid, B_6, and B_{12}, along with a reduction of methionine-rich animal protein foods should be incorporated immediately into the diet if homocysteine levels are high. Follow-up testing should be performed periodically to monitor homocysteine levels and adjust vitamin and dietary therapy.

Ferritin

This is a protein in blood plasma called an iron-binding protein. It is the primary storage form of iron in the body. The measurable level of ferritin corresponds with the body's stores of iron. Higher than normal levels pose two risks for cardiovascular health. First, high values are associated with inflammatory disease. Second, excess ferritin can easily become the target of free radicals, oxidize, and become very dangerous to the cardiovascular system.

Normal values are as follows: men—15 to 300 ng/ul (nanograms per microliter); women—12 to 150 ng/ul.

Glucose—Fasting Blood Sugar

This test simply measures the level of glucose in your blood at the time the blood is drawn. It is usually taken after you have fasted for eight to twelve hours. This assures a reading that is not altered by glucose released by food. Its purpose is to detect any abnormalities in blood sugar levels that would indicate diabetes, hypoglycemia, hyperglycemia, or other dysglycemias (blood sugar disorders) resulting from an inability of the pancreas to produce insulin, a reduced number of insulin receptors, the inability of the intestines to absorb glucose, or the inability of liver to break down glycogen.

Normal values: fasting—70 to 110 mg/dl; nonfasting—under age fifty, 70 to 115 mg/dl; over age fifty, 85 to 125mg/dl.

Although this is a good general screening test, it only measures a momentary level of glucose at the time the blood was drawn. The HbA1c—glycohemoglobin test is a significantly more accurate evaluation of overall blood sugar status and should be performed whether there are blood sugar problems or not.

Hba1c—Glycohemoglobin

This test measures glycohemoglobin, a minor form of hemoglobin found in blood. Hemoglobin (A1) undergoes glycosylation (attachment to glucose), in a slow process within the red blood cells during a 90- to 120-day period. The red blood cell combines with some glucose in the blood. Glucose attaches to the oxygen and iron transporting protein, hemoglobin, in the red blood cell. The amount of glucose that the red blood cell stores depends on how much glucose is available in the blood over the 90- to 120-day period. It reveals how many red blood cells have glucose attached to them during their 90- to 120-day life cycle. This gives an average reading of blood sugar during the three- to four-month period prior to the test and is a much better indicator of overall glucose status than the momentary measurement of glucose taken in the standard blood panel. Results are expressed as a percentage of the total hemoglobin value. Normal values: 4.0 percent to 7.0 percent; 7.0 percent+ indicates a diabetic status.

By contrast to the glucose test, this one is not affected by time of day, meal intake, exercise, drugs, or stress.

Lipid Profile

This group of blood tests measures circulating values for lipids, blood fats such as total cholesterol, LDL cholesterol, VLDL cholesterol, HDL cholesterol, and triglycerides. After the values are compiled, the laboratory establishes a ratio between total cholesterol and HDL, which is somewhat indicative of the risk of cardiovascular heart disease.

Total Cholesterol

This test measures the combination of LDL, HDL, and VLDL cholesterols. Normal range: 140 to 220 mg/dl.

This normal range is way too broad. Hundreds of thousands of people with "normal" cholesterol levels have heart attacks and strokes. Although we know that cholesterol is not the only nor the best predictor of heart disease, elevated levels are reasonably indicative of some metabolic imbalance, which can lead to coronary artery disease.

A safer normal range for cardiovascular health is 150 to 175 mg/dl.

LDL Cholesterol

This is a measurement of low-density lipoprotein, which carries fats from the liver throughout the body. Excess LDL is associated with the development of heart disease.

Normal ranges: Less than 130 mg/dl is normal. 130 to 159 is considered borderline high. 160+ is high risk. This "normal" is too high. To achieve a total cholesterol level of 150 to 175, this value should be less than 100 mg/dl.

HDL Cholesterol

This is a measurement of high-density lipoprotein that removes LDL cholesterol from tissues and brings it back via blood to the liver for breakdown. Normal range: 35 to 70 mg/dl for men and 35 to 85 mg/dl for women.

Once again, this range is too broad. A healthier normal range is 50 to 70 mg/dl. A higher risk of cardiovascular disease is associated with levels in the less than 50 mg/dl range. Levels below 35 mg/dl tell us that very little LDL is being taken back to the liver for breakdown and is a strong indicator of potential cardiovascular damage.

The ratio that is used as a predictor of heart disease is total cholesterol divided by HDL cholesterol. For example:

Total cholesterol = 200
HDL cholesterol = 50
Ratio of total cholesterol to HDL cholesterol,
    200 divided by 50 = 4 to 1

What the ratios mean:

- 3 to 1 or below: low cardiovascular disease/accident risk
- 3 to 1 to 4 to 1: mild cardiovascular disease/accident risk
- 4 to 1 to 5 to 1: moderate cardiovascular disease/accident risk
- 5 to 1 and higher: high cardiovascular disease/accident risk

These values and risk ratios are important to consider, but at this point we know that they hardly paint anywhere near the whole risk picture.

Triglycerides

These are the fats circulating in your blood and represent 90 to 95 percent of fat stored in fat cells. Normal range: men—40 to 160 mg/dl; women—35 to 135 mg/dl.

Levels above 125 mg/dl are considered a risk factor for cardiovascular disease because they indicate excess fats circulating in the blood that can become oxidized and attach to artery walls. Triglycerides thicken the blood, which reduces the flow of oxygen and nutrients to cells. Triglycerides also impair insulin function and raise blood sugar.

Blood Pressure

This noninvasive test measures the pressure of oxygen-rich blood against the artery walls when the heart pumps it out (systolic pressure—upper number) at the peak of the pumping cycle. It also measures the lowest pressure of blood against the artery walls when the heart rests in between beats (diastolic pressure—lower number). Elevated blood pressure is a major risk factor for cardiovascular damage, cardiovascular accidents, fatal heart attacks, and strokes. While both numbers are important, the diastolic resting blood pressure is considered more important in the diagnosis of hypertension, while the systolic pressure is considered a strong indicator of CVD risk. Normal ranges are as follows:

- Normal blood pressure is 120 (systolic—upper number) over 80 (diastolic—lower number).
- Borderline high blood pressure range is 120 to 160 over 90 to 94.

- Mild high range is 140 to 160 over 95 to 104.
- Moderate high range is 140 to 180 over 105 to 114.
- Severe high range is 160+ over 115+

One measurement of blood pressure in the doctor's office every six months or every year, assuming you go that often, is not a clear indication of whether hypertension exists. White Coat Syndrome, which occurs when the stress of the doctor visit increases blood pressure above your normal range, can be quite misleading. Purchasing a blood pressure monitor and taking your own readings at home can provide an accurate determination of blood pressure.

Heart Rate

This simple test measures the number of times that your heart beats (pumps blood out into the circulatory system) in a one-minute period. Chronically slow heart rates (bradychardia) as well as elevated heart rates (tachychardia) are indicative of an underactive or overactive heart from a variety of causes. It is easy to learn how to measure your pulse on your wrist or carotid artery.

Pulse Oximetry

This noninvasive test measures the percentage of oxygen saturation in your blood against an ideal saturation level of 100 percent, indicating how much oxygen is available for cellular metabolism.

Clotting, Fibrinogen, and Prothrombin (PT) Time

This test is considered one of the most important for determining how the blood coagulates. It measures the clotting ability of five plasma coagulation factors. They are prothrombin (the precursor to thrombin that is produced in your liver), which the body uses in conjunction with vitamin K to clot the blood; fibrinogen; factor V; factor VII; and factor X. Measurement of what is called the prothrombin time tells you how quickly your blood clots. A ten- to fourteen-second clotting time is considered normal. Clotting times that are lengthy can mean unnecessary bleeding, particularly if the injury is internal, especially in cardiovascular vessels. This can lead to a hemorrhagic stroke.

Platelet Aggregation

When there is an injury to a blood vessel wall, the body initiates the repair mechanism that we discussed in the chapter on the clotting factor. Platelets collect and aggregate to form a plug at the injury site with the help of fibrinogen and substances that initiate platelet formation, such as the stress hormone epinephrine, arachadonic acid (an omega-6 fatty acid), collagen, and thrombin. Excessive platelet aggregation (stickiness) can give off potent compounds that accelerate the formation of plaque. Platelets can also form clots that stick in small arteries and can impede blood flow, causing angina, a heart attack, or stroke. This test determines whether platelets in blood are clumping together too much, too aggressively, or insufficiently.

CRP: C-Reactive Protein

This blood test measures a special protein that is manufactured in the liver and circulates in the blood at very low levels, typically 3 to 9 nanograms per milliliter in healthy people. C-reactive protein levels rise in the blood when inflammation due to tissue destruction and/or infection, or any disease or condition that brings about inflammation is present, indicating that an above-normal level of inflammation exists. This is an antigen-antibody reaction test that is nonspecific for measuring the severity and course of inflammatory disease and conditions in which there is tissue necrosis (death), such as heart attack, arterial injury, malignancies, and rheumatoid arthritis. Elevated levels of CRP can be detected in the blood eighteen to twenty-four hours after the onset of tissue damage.

Normal range: less than 0.8 mg/dl. More than .08 mg/dl suggests a cause of inflammation that should be investigated further by the doctor and treated nutritionally with systemic oral enzymes.

Electrocardiogram (EKG or ECG)

This test is a printable recording of the electrical impulses that stimulate the heart to contract and can be measured at the surface of your skin. It also indicates cardiac dysfunction that affects the ability of the heart muscle to beat and pump correctly. It can diagnose irregular heart rhythms, interruptions of blood flow, heart attacks, the position and size of the heart, enlargement of heart chambers, inflammation of heart muscle, or delays of electrical impulses. This is a good diagnostic test to uncover a number of cardiac abnormalities and should be taken as part of an annual physical.

Exercise Stress Test

This is an electrocardiogram that is administered while you are walking on a treadmill, steadily increasing your heart rate from the resting rate to the maximum rate.

Echocardiogram

This noninvasive test is a sonogram of the heart. It records the position, size, shape, and movement of the heart valves and chamber walls. The Doppler echocardiogram can also record the movement of blood and shows the velocity of blood flow and the amount of blood, called the ejection fraction, that the heart pumps with each beat. It can detect leakage from valves or the sac around the heart (pericardium). Echocardiograms work by aiming high-frequency sound waves at the heart to locate and record movements by recording echoes. This is accomplished because sound can easily travel through fluids like blood.

There is no pain or discomfort while taking this thirty- to forty-five-minute test that can diagnose a variety of heart irregularities.

Ultrafast CT Scan

This is also known as a computerized axial tomography (CAT) scan, a high-speed computed tomography study that uses X rays similar to conventional ones. It has a scanner that gives rapid, complex calculations of multiple X-ray beams that are not absorbed by tissue in its path. The Ultrafast CT is a fast, noninvasive test that scans the heart and coronary vessels to determine the level and development of atherosclerosis by measuring the level and rate of calcification of arterial plaques, considered strong indicators of atherosclerosis.

Get Tested Regularly

If the values obtained from blood tests are normal, they should ideally be repeated every six months but not less than once per year. Carotid artery palpation should be performed by the doctor at each semiannual or annual exam, along with blood pressure and heart rate tests. You should be monitoring your heart rate and blood pressure weekly on your own at home. Electrocardiogram and/or exercise stress tests should be taken yearly, along with an echocardiogram. The Ultrafast CT scan should be done once after age forty to establish a baseline and again every three years after that. If cardiovascular disease exists, the test should be repeated yearly. Pulse oximetry is recommended once per year. When test values are not normal, they should be repeated every three months or less, according to your physician's advice.

PART II

The Mechanics of Cardio Destruction

To CLEARLY AND SIMPLY UNDERSTAND HOW CARDIOVASCULAR disease and the threat of heart attacks or stroke become a sad reality for millions of unsuspecting Americans each year, we need to take a close, careful look at the biochemical, physiological, neurological, electrical, and nutritional mechanics of destruction in the cardiovascular system. We have termed this *cardiodestruction*.

However, in this discussion we must acknowledge the body's innate heredity ability to seek balance on both a metabolic and physiological level. This striving for balance is called *homeostasis* and it involves thousands of chemical activities in the metabolic pathways. And so while internal and external factors work to erode the cardiovascular system, the Cardiovascular Metabolic Repair Response (CMRR) works to bring your body back to fully functioning health.

In our investigation we'll look at the following:

- How vitamin C deficiency creates an absence or deficiency of collagen that results in the formation of weak artery walls subject to injury, lesions, other damages, inflammation, initiation of CMRR, and the immune system response.
- How cholesterol first works as a "patch and plug" molecule for the artery wall, then as a plaque initiator and collector, joining lipoprotein(a) in CMRR that first repairs arterial lesions and promotes the atherosclerotic process.
- How lipoprotein(a), the adhesive lipoprotein, is a biological Dr. Jekyll and Mr. Hyde that first works as a "patch and plug" repair molecule that initiates CMRR, then works as a plaque initiator and collector that promotes the atherosclerotic process.
- How homocysteine, a nonessential amino acid in the form of homocysteine thiolactone, destroys artery linings and initiates CMRR that, in turn, promotes the atherosclerotic process.
- How insulin erodes arterial linings *and* initiates CMRR that promotes the atherosclerotic process.
- How glucose from sugars and excess refined carbohydrates attaches to proteins in the arterial wall in a process called "glycation" to form Advanced Glycation End Substances (AGES) that destroy arterial linings and initiate CMRR that promotes the atherosclerotic process.
- How EFA deficiency lets down the guard on cell membranes and sets the stage for an unhealthy exchange of nutrients, oxygen, and wastes, causing elevated blood pressure and rigid arteries that rupture easily.
- How arterial inflammation causes an immune system response that brings unwanted cells to the artery wall and starts CMRR, which promotes the atherosclerotic process.
- How chronically elevated adrenalin levels erode artery walls and initiate CMRR that promotes the atherosclerotic process.

- How the immune system responds to arterial injury and the systemic inflammation it causes, cleaning up the mess by initiating CMRR that promotes the atherosclerotic process.
- How the clotting factors, fibrinogen, fibrin, plasminogen, plasmin, and t-PA (tissue plasminogen) provide an emergency CMRR system that can prevent fatal heart attacks and strokes and then promotes the atherosclerotic process.
- How free radical damage aggressively irritates, injures, and destroys arterial linings and initiates CMRR that promotes the atherosclerotic process.
- How obesity stresses the heart; how congenital defects prevent smooth heart operation; how bacterial dental infections irritate, injure, and destroy arterial linings; how overexertion stresses the heart; how smoking, alcohol, and drugs irritate, injure, and destroy arterial linings, all initiating the Cardiovascular Metabolic Repair Response.

Vitamin C Deficiency:
The Overlooked Culprit

E IGHTEENTH-CENTURY BRITISH SAILORS—"LIMEYS"—ATE LIMES and solved the mystery of scurvy and unknowingly, heart disease. Scurvy is an early stage of atherosclerosis and a telltale sign of impending death.

You're probably wondering what all this mumbo jumbo has to do with treating heart disease. As you'll soon see, more than you can imagine. Thanks to the wonders of medical anthropology, we can understand what man was like physiologically, biochemically, and genetically thousands, even hundreds of thousands of years ago.

Thanks to the revolutionary lifesaving investigative work of worldrenowned cardiologist and researcher, Matthias Rath, M.D., and the biochemical genius of the late, great, two-time Nobel Prize winner Linus Pauling, Ph.D., we know that chronic vitamin C deficiency, coupled with lipoprotein(a) deposits, is an independent risk factor far more significant than cholesterol in the development of cardiovascular disease. In 1994, Drs. Pauling and Rath patented a therapy for cardiovascular disease. At that time, Linus Pauling, considered one of the twenty great minds of the twentieth century, made this statement in a *British Journal of Optimum Nutrition* interview, "Now I've gotten to the point where I think we can get almost complete control of cardiovascular disease, heart attacks, and strokes."

In support of that, Dr. Rath, Dr. Pauling's research partner and author of *Eradicating Heart Disease*, believes "all blood risk factors known today in clinical cardiology can be neutralized by vitamin C and other essential nutrients, like lysine, proline, niacin (nicotinic acid form), l-carnitine, and coenzyme Q10."

We emphatically agree!

Unfortunately, the work of these two geniuses has been largely ignored and summarily dismissed again and again as inconclusive. This is a serious misunderstanding of the evidence! Before Dr. Pauling's death in 1994 at age ninety-three, he and Dr. Rath established the connection among vitamin C deficiency, a compromised arterial system, and the development of atherosclerosis. The overwhelming evidence is staring the medical and scientific communities in the face. Yet they choose to discredit and ignore it. Why? Are they afraid to truly heal, protect, and cure mankind from this epidemic health scourge that eventually kills every other person? Are the pharmaceutical companies and the government setting it aside because of pressure?

We have known for some time that atherosclerosis is unquestionably a vitamin C deficiency disease. And it has been known since 1973, thanks to the discovery that was the hypothesis and the major premise of the 1985 Brown-Goldstein Nobel Prize in Medicine, that atherosclerotic plaques form on the linings of artery walls in response to blood vessel injury.

In 1973, Dr. Joseph L. Goldstein, Chief of Molecular Genetics, and Dr. Michael S. Brown, Director of the Department of Genetic Disease at the University of Texas Health Science Center in Dallas, discovered how LDL receptors in the body pull LDL cholesterol out of the blood. According to their revolutionary work, about 70 percent of LDL receptors lie on the surface of liver cells. When too little cholesterol is removed from the blood because of defective LDL receptors, or there are too few of them, cholesterol builds up in the blood and forms plaque on artery walls.

They further suggested that only about 5 percent of people have inherited defects of LDL receptors, commenting that many people develop deficiencies of LDL receptors as a result of the Standard American Diet (SAD). Goldstein and Brown claim that high-fat, high-cholesterol diets lead to suppression of LDL receptors because they trick the cells into thinking there is plenty of cholesterol and additional receptors are not necessary. This is extremely dangerous because cholesterol is not removed from blood fast enough and can transform into oxidized LDL cholesterol that aggressively attaches to artery walls, becoming a major risk factor for atherosclerosis.

A Damage and Repair Theory Based on Genetic Intelligence

Human beings were initially programmed genetically to produce vitamin C in the liver by employing four enzymes to convert it from glucose. Noted vitamin C expert Dr. Irwin Stone, author of *The Healing Factor: Vitamin C Against Disease*, believes "[we] can surmise that the production of ascorbic acid was an early accomplishment of the life process because of its wide distribution in nearly all present-day living organisms. It is produced in comparatively large amounts in the simplest plants and the most complex; it is synthesized in the most primitive animal species as well as in the most highly organized. Except possibly for a few microorganisms, those species of animals that cannot make their own ascorbic acid are the exceptions and require it in their food if they are to survive. Without it, life cannot exist. Because of its nearly universal presence in both plants and animals we can assume that its production was well organized before the time when evolving life forms diverged along separate plant and animal lines."

According to the unprecedented medical anthropology discovery made by Dr. Rath, the former first Director of Cardiovascular Research at the Linus Pauling Institute of Science and Medicine, man lost his ability thousands of generations ago to manufacture 1-gulonolactone oxidase, one of four enzymes necessary to produce vitamin C internally. He stated that vitamin C in the blood is very low in humans; consequently, lipoprotein(a) and heart disease are high. Conversely, vitamin C is high in animals because it is produced endogenously (internally) on demand. As a result, lipoprotein(a) is low or nonexistent and the same is true for heart disease! Biochemist Dr. Irwin Stone tells us that this occurred about sixty million years ago.[1]

The metabolic process of internal vitamin C production went awry then and one enzyme became defective. As an unfortunate result, prehistoric man could no longer produce vitamin C on demand. Losing this ability halted the spontaneous, immediate production and supply of vitamin C in our livers according to our complex, ever-changing metabolic needs. Man had to then obtain vitamin C from nutritional sources in food.

This deficiency did not initially present a problem since our ancestral prehistoric hunter-gatherers were able to get enough vitamin C from the fresh fruits, berries, and vegetables and other plant foods they found. During the Ice Ages, of which there were several, global temperatures dropped. Data from the last Ice Age, four hundred to five hundred generations ago, show that man received very little food, was close to starvation, and obtained practically no vitamins.

The onset of the Ice Ages severely restricted the ability of all types of vitamin C-rich foods, such as fruits and vegetables, to flourish. There were virtually no sources to be found. Without sufficient amounts of essential vitamin C for thousands of years, people's arteries did not develop enough collagen to make them healthy and strong. Production of collagen, the connective tissue that holds our bodies together, was barely possible and the collagen our ancestors produced was deformed and unable to form strong, resistant, fibrous masses.

Without healthy collagen, arteries lose their natural thickness, density, and flexibility. They become porous and leaky. Then they cannot resist the pressure of blood pumping and surging through them sixty or more times per minute. Weak and constantly bombarded with pressure, they rupture. On the outside, easy bruising in large patches occurs. Even the slightest touch can cause many small capillaries to break, causing bruises. Capillaries and small arteries in the nose begin to rupture and bloody noses are common. Anal capillaries frequently break, causing rectal bleeding. Hemorrhages in larger arteries cause blood to leak into the body. This prevents the blood from delivering the critical supply of oxygen and nutrients to cells, while removing metabolic wastes. Coronary arteries around the heart rupture and starve the heart of its share. Finally, the cardiovascular system breaks down and death is imminent.

As this metabolic scenario occurred over thousands of years, the body's innate ability to heal itself came into play. Via genetic intelligence, adaptation, and modification, man developed a system that used genetic repair molecules to prevent the breakdown of blood vessels. The remedy was a patch and plug system that used lipoprotein(a), cholesterol, and other fats as mortarlike filler substances. Lipoprotein(a), because of its additional sticky molecule, is very effective. Lipoprotein(a) was formed in the liver in greater amounts as a way of repairing the devastating damage caused to arteries by vitamin C deficiency. Those who passed on the gene for lipoprotein(a) survived, and those who did not perished. Now, as it was then, lipoprotein(a) is the solution to the problem. But at the same time it repairs the arterial wall damage, it causes the problem of plaque formation.

Among the vitamin deficiencies of our ancestors, vitamin C was the greatest. And that vitamin C deficiency, known as scurvy, often resulted in death caused by massive blood loss resulting from the inability to produce collagen. Bleeding gums was a visible sign of scurvy that was evidenced by sailors of earlier centuries. Vitamin C, scarce for thousands of generations, was a prominent threat to human existence.[2,3] Humans needed to develop repair mechanisms and they did. Lipoprotein(a), other fat-transporting particles like LDL cholesterol, and clotting factors were the body's way of compensating. The genetic information required to produce these repair molecules was passed down from generation to generation. Prior to that, man, like most living species, produced vitamin C in the liver from molecules of sugar, anywhere from 1,000 to 20,000 mg per day, for collagen production and repair, antioxidant activity, and other metabolic functions. Thousands of researchers, doctors, nutritionists, and biochemistry educators are convinced that vitamin C deficiency is the number one cause of heart disease.

Because of vitamin C's primary function of manufacturing collagen, its absence in the blood results in the inability to produce collagen and has a major impact on the way other causative factors come into play.

> Chronic vitamin C deficiency causes two major problems: artery wall instability (scurvy) and artery wall lesions (injuries).

Cells that separate the artery orifice (lumen) from the arterial lining (endothelial cells) become unstable and leaky. When vitamin C is scarce in the blood, the stage is set for damage, initiating the Cardiovascular Metabolic Repair Response and the development of atherosclerosis. When the walls come tumbling down, it's metabolic annihilation for the arteries!

Chronic Vitamin C Deficiency and Subclinical Scurvy Syndrome (SSS)

Sounds confusing, but it's not. Chronic vitamin C deficiency is common in humans because, as we learned earlier, we cannot produce vitamin C on demand internally like most other mammals. When vitamin

C is lacking in our diets, which means it is lacking internally for essential metabolic processes, a condition called scurvy develops. This usually occurs when intake is less than 50 milligrams of vitamin C per day for even just a few months.

Bleeding gums, nosebleeds, easy bruising, and broken skin are common symptoms that warrant a visit to your nutritionally naive doctor. He will not even remotely think this is scurvy and consequently not consider vitamin C deficiency as the cause. When these symptoms occur, we call it subclinical scurvy syndrome (SSS). SSS causes arteries and capillaries to become weak throughout the cardiovascular system. Wherever there is a weak, defectively developed collagen matrix that ruptures, arterial injury results. The symptoms we see and experience are warning signs of a more serious problem existing in the cardiovascular system that many of us unknowingly have. SSS and scurvy are clear signs of cardiovascular disease.

Scurvy: It's Still a Scourge

Vitamin C was actually discovered in 1928, when Nobel Prize winner Albert von Szent-Gyorgyi, M.D., Ph.D., isolated a substance (hexuronic acid) that was identical to vitamin C. He proposed the name ascorbic acid. Interestingly, *ascorbic* means "without scurvy" in Latin.

While it is obvious that most of us in the Western world don't display symptoms of scurvy in any visible sense, most of us do internally. On the mild side, the chronic bleeding of gums and nosebleeds are clear signs of vitamin C deficiency and SSS. Most important, atherosclerosis is an invisible form of scurvy. We cannot see it from the outside; there are no painful symptoms, just constant small breaks and ruptures in artery walls that the body silently repairs with lipoprotein(a) and cholesterol that keep building up with each successive injury, forming dangerous plaques that break off and cause heart attacks and strokes.

The Vitamin C–Heart Disease Connection: How Long Have We Known?

Thousands of positive research studies about vitamin C have been conducted and published in peer-reviewed medical and scientific journals by world-renowned experts. An endless amount of empirical (practice-based) evidence, plus patents issued for vitamin C in cardiovascular care, support its effectiveness. Despite that, information is difficult to find in health care and medical textbooks, courses, or programs about the natural, cardiovascular, antioxidant, and therapeutic whole-body benefits of vitamin C. It seems purposely overlooked.

According to Emanuel Cheraskin, M.D., D.M.D., coauthor of *The Vitamin C Connection*, "there are more than ten thousand published scientific papers that make it quite clear that there is not one body process (such as what goes on inside cells or tissues) and not one disease or syndrome (from the common cold to leprosy) that is not influenced—directly or indirectly—by vitamin C." Cardiovascular disease is no exception!

The Collagen Connection

The word *collagen* originated from the Greek "to produce glue." A deficiency of collagen is an early stage of atherosclerosis caused primarily by a deficiency of vitamin C, lysine, and proline.

What is collagen? Collagen is the major building block protein in your body. It is the glue or ground substance among cells that connects and holds tissues, organs, and bones together. It is a rigid, fibrous protein that is the principal substance in the connective tissue of animals. Without collagen you would literally fall apart. Scientifically, the term *collagen* refers to a group of building-block proteins with a fibrous structure that are capable of forming insoluble fibers that possess great strength.

- It is the most abundant protein in mammals.

- It is the major fibrous element of blood vessels, skin, bone, intervertebral discs, tendons, cartilage, ligaments, teeth, the cornea, and the eye lens.
- It is present in all organs.
- It is involved in the formation of newly developing tissue.

Without vitamin C, it is possible for the body to produce a small amount of collagen. However, the collagen that is synthesized in this way will not be of normal, healthy, cross-linked fiber structure. Deformed collagen, structurally weaker and more leaky than the healthy variety, leads to severe fragility of arteries, veins, capillaries, and microcapillaries that cause nosebleeds, bleeding gums, hemorrhoidal bleeding, and easy bruising. These are early warning signs, characteristic of scurvy, that are indicative of other injured, damaged, or ruptured blood vessels, such as coronary arteries, that have developed atherosclerosis.

The most prevalent kind of collagen in the body is Type I, found in skin, tendons, bone, and the cornea. Type II collagen is found in cartilage and intervertebral discs of the spine. Type III collagen is found in the cardiovascular system and fetal skin. Type IV collagen is found in some cell membranes, and Type V collagen is found in placenta and skin.

Our primary interest is in Type III collagen, found in cardiovascular tissue. For the purpose of our discussion it is the most important.

Collagen has a unique and unusual amino acid protein structure that sets it apart from other body–building block proteins. There is more of the amino acid proline in collagen than in most other proteins. Complex derivatives of the amino acids proline (4-hydroxyproline) and lysine (5-hydroxylysine) are major components of collagen, yet are found in few other proteins.

Proline, considered a nonessential amino acid, is the third most heavily concentrated free amino acid in the body fluids of adults. Ample reserves of proline are found and stored in collagen, which makes up about 25 to 30 percent of the body's proteins. Because of its vital role in the production of healthy collagen, proline should be considered essential for health. Proline has the unique ability to replace incomplete and structurally weak collagen residues (lysyl residues) found in arterial connective tissue, helping to strengthen it and prevent arterial injury. That is why proline and lysine are crucial for proper, healthy collagen formation and the structural integrity of the cardiovascular network.

Deficiencies of these amino acids, vitamin C, and/or a deficiency of sulfur prevent necessary amounts of collagen from forming and incorporating into strong, healthy arteries that maintain maximum cardiovascular health. Vitamin B_6 and copper are also essential for the cross-linking of collagen fibers.

How Vitamin C Contributes to a Healthy Heart

Dr. James Enstrom of the University of California at Los Angeles (UCLA) School of Public Health studied more than eleven thousand people over a ten-year period regarding the risk of CVD and vitamin C. The impressive results were heralded by *Newsweek* magazine, the *Los Angeles Times*, and the *New York Times*. The study compared Americans on a typical Standard American Diet, low in vitamin C intake, to those supplementing their diets with 300 mg of vitamin C daily. For those men who consumed the 300 mg from supplements and food, heart disease was cut in half, compared to the Standard American Diet.[4] For those women who consumed the 300 mg from supplements and food, heart disease was cut by one-third, compared to the

> Vitamin C reduces the risk of cardiovascular disease and increases longevity.

Standard American diet.[5] Men taking 150 mg of vitamin C lived two years longer than the central group, and men taking 300 mg of vitamin C lived six years longer. A similar trend was also observed in women.

- Vitamin C helps build a strong, healthy collagen matrix and flexible arteries, and restores blood vessel stability.
- Vitamin C also assists in the efficient metabolism of amino acids. This is important specifically for the cardiovascular system to properly metabolize lysine, proline, and arginine in order to build and cross-link healthy collagen.[6]
- Vitamin C lowers LDL cholesterol levels.
- Vitamin C, synergistically with B_5, controls the production of stress hormones.
- Vitamin C enhances immune system activity.
- Vitamin C also prevents the dangerous proliferation of smooth muscle cells in the intima of the artery.

The Confusion
over Cholesterol

IN 1913, NIKOLAI ANITSHKOW, A RUSSIAN SCIENTIST, WAS THE first to give cholesterol a bad rap. After feeding rabbits a high-cholesterol diet, he examined their blood vessels and found they were hardened and clogged with plaque. From that crude study, he concluded that cholesterol caused heart disease. In one respect he was right, as cholesterol is one of the body's two prime substances called out to repair arterial injury. Believe it when we tell you that cholesterol is your friend. The health benefits of cholesterol far outweigh its dangers. And cholesterol will remain your friend as long as you treat your body right with health-promoting food, specifically sufficient quantities of essential fatty acids.

The Misunderstanding

Cholesterol is probably one of the most misunderstood substances in the human body. It belongs to a group of fatty, waxlike substances called sterols (thus chole-sterol) that is produced only in the liver of animals and not by any plants. That's right, there is no cholesterol in fruits, vegetables, nuts, seeds, and grains—none! Cholesterol has continually been given a really bad rap over the years by the medical, health, and pharmaceutical communities. However, it is undeniably essential for life and health.

Here are cholesterol's five main functions:

1. Cholesterol is an essential component of all cell membranes and a major building block of body tissues. All cell membranes in the body constantly require it, along with EFAs, to maintain their elasticity. It regulates the traffic of nutrients, water, and oxygen into the cells. At the same time it carries metabolic wastes, toxins, and carbon dioxide out of the cells. We tend to forget that LDL, widely considered the "bad" cholesterol, is the medium in which fat-soluble antioxidants, such as vitamin E and carotenoids, transport themselves through the blood for metabolic processes in cells and tissues.

2. Cholesterol is the essential first step in the production of many hormones. Certain glands, like the adrenals and the pancreas, use cholesterol to manufacture steroid or cortisone-like hormones (including sex hormones) that control many functions in the body.

3. Cholesterol is also crucial to vitamin D synthesis under the skin. Without cholesterol we can't make any vitamin D, which is critical for bone development. Without vitamin D, we cannot build healthy bones, regenerate new bone, or maintain bone mass.

4. Cholesterol assists the liver in producing bile acids that are essential to the digestion of fats in the small intestine and to the detoxification of poisons.

5. Although cholesterol is an essential substance for many metabolic processes, it also becomes a "Mr. Fix-It" response

and repair mechanism for damaged arteries. Problems with cholesterol arise when too much of it is produced, allowing it to adhere to artery walls, or when it oxidizes (biologically rusts), adhering much more readily, and collecting hard mineral deposits, such as calcium circulating in the arteries. Excess cholesterol fills up macrophages from the immune system to form foam cells. This chokes the cells, and cholesterol leaks out into developing plaques.

LDL cholesterol is a prime target of free radical oxidation. There is much in the literature showing that various changes in LDL cholesterol significantly increases its ability to cause hardening of the arteries; this ability is known as atherogenicity. When LDL cholesterol does not contain sufficient levels of antioxidants, it becomes prone to oxidation. Therefore, high levels of oxidized LDL cholesterol are recognized as an early step in the development of coronary artery disease (CAD).

- Oxidized LDL cholesterol has been identified in atherosclerotic lesions.
- Oxidized LDL cholesterol is taken up more readily by macrophages than native (unaltered, as produced by the liver) LDL cholesterol, creating foam cells.
- Oxidized LDL cholesterol is cytotoxic (caustic, irritating) to endothelial cells and may increase vasoconstriction in arteries. Dr. Steinberg, at the Division of Endocrinology and Metabolism, Department of Medicine, University of California, San Diego, tells us that the susceptibility of LDL to oxidation is directly related to the severity of atherosclerosis.[1]

The correlation between oxidized LDL cholesterol and athero-sclerosis was also supported in a study of thirty-five heart attack survivors. Jan Regnstrim, M.D., of the famed Karolinska Hospital and Institute, Stockholm, Sweden, was the principal investigator. Rengstrom studied the susceptibility of LDL cholesterol to oxidation.

He noted a strong association among the severity of premature coronary atherosclerosis, hardening of the arteries, and LDL cholesterol oxidation, suggesting the use of antioxidant supplements to neutralize free radical oxidation of the LDL cholesterol and reduce the risk of coronary artery disease.[2]

Because cholesterol is an oil-like, fatty substance, it does not mix with a water-based fluid such as blood. So, inside the liver, it gets wrapped inside a protein coating, much like meat inside a dumpling, becoming a lipoprotein so that it can travel in the blood.

Cholesterol Movers

Lipoproteins have the job of transporting cholesterol throughout the body. LDLs (low-density lipoproteins) carry cholesterol from the liver to the cells. LDL cholesterol is primarily fat surrounded by a little protein. HDLs (high-density lipoproteins), known to many as the "good" cholesterol, are primarily comprised of protein surrounding a little fat. And with their pocketlike shape, HDLs efficiently carry cholesterol away from artery walls and cells back to the liver for breakdown and excretion. Then there are VLDLs (very low density lipoproteins) manufactured by the liver, precursors to LDL that transport triglycerides. Last, there are chylomicrons, cholesterol-type particles produced by the intestinal walls when fat is digested. Total cholesterol is a combination of LDL, VLDL, and HDL. The ratio of total cholesterol to HDL cholesterol is often used to assess risk of cardiovascular disease.

What Causes High Cholesterol

Though there are many causes of high cholesterol, the five main culprits are as follows:

1. **Cardiovascular accidents:** Whenever there is a cardiovascular accident, from the smallest undetectable injury in an

artery to a large break or rupture that causes a heart attack or stroke, cholesterol is called upon to arrive at the site of the damage and fix it, that is, to patch and plug the area of damage so that the injury does not continue to enlarge or leak. Now you know why cholesterol is your friend in need!

2. **Too few LDL receptors in the liver:** There are thousands of LDL cholesterol receptors in the liver ready and waiting to take back cholesterol circulating in the blood, coming in on HDL cholesterol molecules. Either as a result of genetic predisposition via genetic programming at the time of conception, or due to damage inflicted on the liver for other reasons such as chronic inflammatory status, viral infections like hepatitis, or alcohol-induced cirrhosis, about 5 percent of people are destined to have high cholesterol levels. This occurs because they don't have enough receptors to collect all the returning LDL cholesterol from the blood. Consequently, much more LDL cholesterol will circulate in their blood without a place to land, allowing areas of the artery lining that are not perfectly smooth to attract and pick it up. Researchers involved in the Human Genome project are hard at work analyzing and hopefully understanding the DNA structure of key genes that predispose us to unhealthy conditions such as high cholesterol, cancer, and other disease maladies.

3. **EFA deficiency:** High cholesterol levels in the blood are a clear indication of EFA deficiency. Greater than normal amounts of cholesterol are produced by the liver when there are not enough essential fatty acids in the cell membrane, or the fats on the cell membrane are composed of too many hard, saturated, or trans fats. The body's natural choice is to get the softest fats into the cell membrane. Cholesterol, softer and more flexible than saturated or trans fats, is a softening agent that is better for the cell membrane, although not an ideal fat choice.

4. **Saturated fat:** The main dietary reason that causes cholesterol levels to get out of whack is saturated fat. By their nature and composition, cell membranes ideally have a lot of unsaturated fatty acids on them. This ensures that the membrane is soft, pliable, and flexible to allow the right stuff in and the wrong stuff out. Whenever the cell membrane has too many saturated fatty acids, it seeks to get softer fats to replace the hard ones. This stimulates the liver to produce softer fat for cell membranes. Enter cholesterol, the artery repairman and cell membrane softener. Because cholesterol is softer than saturated or trans fats, it readily takes their place on the cell membrane. Consumption of saturated fat stimulates the production of softer, more artery-friendly substances, such as cholesterol. As this process unfolds and continues with a diet high in saturated fats, cholesterol levels in the blood are correspondingly higher as these fats travel throughout the body as LDL molecules.

5. **Diet:** After carefully studying the literature and research, it appears to us that excess cholesterol in food will raise blood cholesterol to a limited (very limited) extent, but only for a short while, as the liver tightly controls its production.

Is Cholesterol Really Killing You?

It's time to finally explode the "cholesterol causes heart disease" myth. We now know that:

- Cholesterol is essential for life and health.
- Good cholesterol is produced in the liver and tightly controlled.

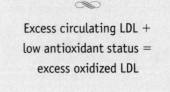

Excess circulating LDL +
low antioxidant status =
excess oxidized LDL

- Cholesterol is needed in all cell membranes throughout the body. It helps regulate what goes in and out of our cells.
- No cholesterol = no hormones. No hormones = no metabolic control!
- You can't have healthy bones without cholesterol.
- Cholesterol is Mr. Fix-It for your arteries, only dispatched and attaching to artery walls when injuries occur.
- Bad cholesterol, oxidized LDL cholesterol, considered extremely dangerous to the cardiovascular system, is the result of too many free radicals and too few antioxidants in the diet.

The Immune System Response

In addition to the bad rap given cholesterol, we must remember that the human body is gifted with an intelligent, intricate system of checks and balances. As our arteries continue to accumulate fat globules of lipoprotein(a) (to be discussed in the next chapter), LDL cholesterol, and other substances, as they age as a result of constant, unrelenting free radical damage, or when they are injured, the immune system sends out a crew of helper cells. These cells clean up areas of plaque along artery walls, preventing further damage.

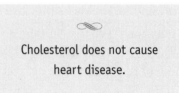

Cholesterol does not cause heart disease.

Macrophage Mania

Repeated injuries to endothelial cells that make up the endothelium stimulate the formation of cell adhesion molecules, called CAMs. CAMs spark a healing and repair process by attaching a biochemical ID tag on the cell. This identifies the enemy and sends a signal for help in the blood vessel network. The immune response causes arterial walls to attract white blood cells called monocytes. These monocytes attach to the blood vessel lining from the immune system. Monocytes squeeze among the endothelial cells, causing inflammation in the tissue below. As previously mentioned, these monocytes convert to macrophages that act like sponges, soaking up cholesterol in the artery. When examined microscopically, the stuffed macrophages have a foamy appearance and are called foam cells. As these foam cells accumulate, they attract more fats, removing them from the artery wall. CAMs and macrophages collect cholesterol, lipoprotein(a), and platelets that travel to the injury site. A protein coating called a fibrous cap forms over the young, growing plaque. Then the macrophages burst and die. Their contents flood out under the fibrous cap into the plaque. This cellular waste destroys and destabilizes the cap. The unstable plaque is vulnerable to increases in blood pressure that can burst it. In many instances these younger plaques become weak, rupture, and form sudden, massive clots that cause a heart attack or stroke.

Some plaques continue to mature by collecting lipoprotein(a), LDL cholesterol, oxidized LDL cholesterol, triglycerides, other fats, and calcium. The deposits begin to harden and calcify, becoming more stiff and inflexible as they grow. Mature and fully developed plaques continue to calcify, harden, and stabilize, and rarely rupture. Eventually, they can occupy 70 percent or more of the potential blood volume of the artery, severely restricting blood flow and causing angina. Or, in the case of a complete blockage, they initiate a debilitating or potentially fatal stroke or heart attack.

There's more. Vitamin C stimulates the production of antibodies, our immune system's line of defense against infectious foreign substances or antigens. A one-year study, conducted in Antarctica by S. Vallance, indicated that beneficial IGGS and IGM antibodies increased with additional vitamin C intake. IGMs are primary antibodies that circulate in blood to kill bacteria.[3]

Simultaneously, the immune system monitors other foreign invaders in the blood that can do arterial damage. Food allergies overwork the immune system. When proteins in food cross the gastrointestinal barrier and enter the blood, a condition known as "leaky gut syndrome," the immune system reacts to them as foreign invaders and begins a seek-and-destroy mission. This activity diverts the immune system away from other protective patrol and kill work. Arterial injury also causes the immune system to divert its energy from other activities so that it can send monocytes to damage sites. These combined activities take vital power away from the ability of the immune system to destroy invading bacterium, viruses, and other pathogens.

SEVEN

Free Radical Damage, Antioxidants, and Heart Disease

OUTSIDE, THE CULTURAL WARS OF THE WORLD THUNDER ON. Within, the biological wars between free radicals and antioxidants have raged on since the beginning of time. Do you know what epigallocatechin is? Or singlet oxygen and peroxynitrite? Ever heard of alpha-lipoic acid and ORACs? This seemingly foreign language is a key to your cardiovascular health. But it doesn't have to be foreign. What are these invisible friends and foes anyway?

Free Radicals: The Enemy Within

Without the right protection, the Tin Man in *The Wizard of Oz* would have rusted away. And without antioxidants protecting us from the relentless attack of free radicals, we would rust on the inside, develop disease, and die young. While practically everyone wants something free, you certainly don't want these.

In 1952, Denham Harmon pioneered the free radical theory of oxidative damage and aging. Free radicals are vicious molecules missing an electron in their outer shells. Most are toxic forms of oxygen molecules. But ironically, oxygen is another nutritional double-edged sword, critical for metabolic processes yet devastating in its reactive forms. These unstable gangsters steal electrons from healthy cells, rendering them "biologically rusted," damaged, or destroyed.

Free radicals spawn from environmental pollution, toxins, pesticides, industrial and household chemicals, sunlight, radiation, food (especially barbecued, charbroiled, or fried foods that produce dangerous nitrosamines when they are cooked), alcohol, smoking, and normal metabolic activity in the body. These injurious free radicals destroy cells, living tissue, and fluids. They rapidly accelerate the aging process, severely damaging the ability of the immune system to battle unwanted pathogens (bacteria, viruses, and parasites) that enjoy invading your body. According to noted American biochemist Dr. Richard Passwater, free radicals are "biological terrorists" of the human terrain.[1]

In much the same way that iron oxidizes and rusts with exposure to the oxygen in air, cells in our body are oxidized or "biologically rusted" by disturbed molecules in our bodies. These molecules are missing a small part called an electron from their outermost shells. That type of molecule, called a "free radical" or pro-oxidant, is extremely active chemically. It tries at all costs to steal its missing electron from a healthy, complete molecule on the cell membrane. In so doing it leaves the cell membrane deficient, destroying it in the process, causing "free radical damage." As large groups of cells are destroyed, areas of tissue are altered, diminishing or ending their ability to function. Tissue necrosis (death of local tissue), diminished metabolic function, and premature aging also occur. But free radical damage doesn't stop there. It causes damage to DNA, your genetic blueprint molecules. This prevents proper replication of healthy cells and accelerates the aging process. The damage occurs continuously when there are large amounts of free radicals circulating as a result of low antioxidant levels or no antioxidants available to neutralize and destroy them. Free radical damage is especially dangerous to arterial tissue and heart muscle. Uncontrolled free radicals in your arteries eat away at the endothelium, then attack the muscle layer underneath. The destruction of arterial tissue in this way causes injuries to form that set the Cardiovascular Metabolic Repair Response into motion.

Jack Challem, of *The Nutrition Reporter*, identifies the most destructive free radicals:[2] hydrogen peroxide, hydroxyl radical, peroxyl radical, singlet oxygen, hypochlorous radical, peroxynitrite radical, and ozone.

Other extremely damaging free radicals found circulating in blood are superoxide, oxidized adrenaline, and lipid peroxides.

Guardians of the Heart and Cardiovascular System

Antioxidants are both nutritive and nonnutritive substances that prevent "free radical" damage to the cells.

- They are free radical scavengers that neutralize and destroy free radicals in cardiovascular tissues, heart muscle, and throughout the body.
- They prevent cell membrane damage that causes tissues to become weak and subject to injury, ensuring the proper flow of nutrients into the cells and the flow of wastes and carbon dioxide out of the cells.
- They prevent the oxidation of fats, particularly LDL cholesterol, considered one of the greatest risk factors for cardiovascular disease.
- They destroy carcinogens.
- They oxygenate the cells, allowing them to process nutrients correctly.

- They stimulate and enhance the activity of immune system function, which provides immune factors in the blood, such as T-cells, NK (natural killer) cells, and macrophages, to combat invading pathogens such as bacteria, viruses, fungi, and toxins derived from food, air, and water.
- They protect against the negative effects of drugs, xenobiotics (foreign substances), toxic metals, volatile petroleum-based fumes, alcohol, cigarette smoke (benzopyrenes and tar), and endogenous (made in the body) pro-oxidant "free radical" substances such as oxidized cholesterol, adrenaline, homocysteine, and oxidized fats.
- They promote the formation of germ-killing enzymes.

Major antioxidants include:

2-O-glycosyl isovitexin
    (barley grass juice)
Alpha-lipoic acid
Astaxanthin
Beta 1,3 glucans
Beta-carotene
Bilberry
Bioflavonoids
Co-enzyme Q10
Cryptoxanthin
Daidzein
D-limonene
EGCG
    (epigallocatechin gallate)
Ellagic acid
Garlic
Genistein
GLA
    (Gamma linolenic acid)

Indole-3-carbinol
Isothiocyanates
L-cysteine
L-gluthathione
L-taurine
Lutein
Lycopene
Melatonin
NAC (n-acetyl cysteine)
Proanthocyanidins
Resveratrol
Selenium
SOD
    (superoxide dismutase)
Sulforaphane
Vitamin A
Vitamin C
Vitamin E
Zeaxanthin

Antioxidants Are Biopolice Working 24/7

As free radical molecules cause oxidation, biological rusting continues inside the body. Antioxidants labor tirelessly to slow down and terminate this oxidation process. These kamikaze lifesaver molecules continually seek and destroy free radicals, sacrificing themselves and self-destructing to save other healthy cells from certain death. Catechins are an example of antioxidants identified in green tea that readily allow themselves to be oxidized in place of more essential molecules in the body.

Some antioxidants, such as the proanthocyanidins found in grape seed and pycnogenol, work to regenerate vitamin C, which then regenerates vitamin E. At the Lipid and Atherosclerosis Prevention Clinic, University of Kansas Medical Center, Kansas City, the prevention of atherosclerosis with antioxidants was supported by the recent research findings of William S. Harris, Ph.D. Because nutrients with antioxidant properties such as vitamin C, vitamin E, and beta-carotene can reduce the susceptibility of LDL (low-density lipoprotein) cholesterol to oxidation, this suggests a role for pharmacologic as well as nutritional antioxidants in the prevention of atherosclerosis.[3]

Dietary antioxidants, such as vitamin E, vitamin C, and beta-carotene, are potent protectors against LDL oxidation. Vitamin E, a fat-soluble antioxidant, is the predominant antioxidant in the LDL cholesterol particle itself. Vitamin C, a water-soluble antioxidant, is thought to be the most effective LDL protector in plasma. A Boston study observed that the group of individuals with the lowest plasma levels of vitamin C tended to have the highest blood pressures. In two other studies, elderly individuals with diets high in vitamin C were least likely to have high blood pressure. In a third study, vitamin C was shown to return oxidized vitamin E back to its original state.

An increase in plasma vitamin C has also been linked to elevated levels of HDL (high-density lipoprotein), the cardioprotective or "good" form of cholesterol. Clinical intervention trials support the cholesterol-lowering effects of vitamin C, although these have not been consistent. Beta-carotene was associated with inhibition of LDL oxidation and the subsequent uptake by macrophages that would occur.[4]

Plants and Antioxidant Action

The plant kingdom is home to an unlimited array of body-friendly antioxidants identified by botanists, biologists, and biochemists. Thousands, perhaps millions more yet unknown, wait to be discovered. Appropriately dubbed "phytonutrients" (*phyto* meaning plant), these nutrients have unfamiliar names such as bioflavonoids, polyphenols, carotenoids, and anthocyanidins.

The Power of Color

Bioflavonoids, the major phytonutrients in foods, are pigments that endow fruits and veggies with their unique and vibrant colors. These pigments are powerful antioxidants. Beta-carotene, an orange bioflavonoid found in yellow to red plant foods, scavenges free radicals and transforms into vitamin A in the liver as needed. Lycopene, a red bioflavonoid, is found in tomatoes, watermelons, and pink grapefruit. Chlorophyll, a green bioflavonoid, is found in green leafy vegetables, cereal grasses, and marine vegetation, such as spirulina, blue green algae, wakame, dulse, and kelp.

Not All Antioxidants Are Phytonutrients

Melatonin, a popular hormone, is produced in the pineal gland situated inside the brain. Studied for its ability to induce sleep and reduce the effects of jet lag, melatonin is possibly the most effective antioxidant in the body, vigorously wiping out hydroxyl radicals. Melatonin is a hidden antioxidant star.

Don't Forget These Antioxidants

The antiaging antioxidant ellagic acid is found in grapes, wine, berries, walnuts, apples, tea, and pomegranates. Bilberry is rich in blue-colored polyphenols that have exceptional antioxidant activity in the eyes. Pycnogenol is an anthocyanidin found in the bark of the Maritime pine tree. D-limonene is found in citrus oils. Epigallocatechin gallate (EGCG), plentiful in green tea, is reported to be two hundred times more potent than vitamin E and perhaps more potent than any other antioxidant.

Stayin' Alive with PhytoFood ORACs

Antioxidants are gifted with the unique ability to latch on to and destroy free radicals. Breakthrough research at the USDA Human Nutrition Center for Aging at Tufts University in Boston, conducted by Ronald Prior, Ph.D., uncovered and evaluated the specific free radical–absorbing capacity of fruits and vegetables.[5,6] This powerful capacity to absorb and neutralize free radicals was measured by Dr. Prior in ORAC units (Oxygen Radical Absorbance Capacity).[7] Specifically, this tells us how aggressively antioxidants in fruits or vegetables destroy free radicals circulating throughout the body and how they effectively prevent cell damage and aging. Eat and drink them every day!

A Fountain of Youth

It's no secret that the French don't slouch when it comes to eating high-fat foods, guzzling perhaps more wine than any culture in the world, and smoking. Yet for years, significantly lower occurrence of heart disease in France compared to the United States remained a mystery. Some experts call it the "French paradox." Wine appears to dramatically lessen the incidence of heart attack and heart disease, and experts cite cardiovascular protection from its regular consumption.

There's much more to it than that. Solid research indicates phytonutrients in the wine, *not* the alcohol, are the awesome antioxidant workers. Red wine and its nonalcoholic equal, purple Concord grape juice, are brimming with the antioxidants resveratrol, grapeseed anthocyanidins, quercetin, ellagic acid, phenolic flavonoids, and epicatechin. Purple Concord grape juice is perhaps the most powerful antioxidant food on earth, having demonstrated the highest ORAC rating of more than forty fruits, vegetables, and juices tested in the lab!

The much talked about antioxidants are the "friendly police" molecules. They give a readily available electron to free radical molecules in order to spare other healthy cells in the body that would otherwise be destroyed.

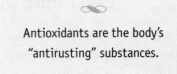

Antioxidants are the body's "antirusting" substances.

Other Physiological Factors

Lipoprotein(a): A Metabolic Dr. Jekyll and Mr. Hyde

The human body makes use of special molecules to deliver essential cholesterol and fat molecules to cells throughout the body. These molecules are called lipoproteins. They are proteins that surround the cholesterol or fats so that they are capable of flowing easily in the blood. Familiar lipoproteins are low-density lipoprotein (LDL) and high-density lipoprotein (HDL). Less familiar but far more important when it comes to cardiovascular disease is lipoprotein(a).

The "Adhesive" Lipoprotein

Called the adhesive lipoprotein, lipoprotein(a) is a metabolic offshoot of low-density lipoprotein cholesterol that first works as a "patch and plug" molecule to repair arterial damage. Then it remains at the damaged site, becoming a plaque initiator and magnet. By attracting, collecting, and accumulating fats and fatlike substances such as cholesterol and triglycerides, minerals such as calcium, and other substances from the blood onto the artery wall, it takes them out of circulation and incorporates itself into the plaque.

According to Dr. Rath's book, *Eradicating Heart Disease*, a variation of LDL cholesterol is produced when a very sticky "adhesive" molecule called apoprotein(a) attaches to it, forming lipoprotein(a). Lipoprotein(a) is a molecule made up of the protein portion of LDL, called apo(b), and another protein called apo(a). These very sticky lipoprotein(a) molecules easily adhere to the artery wall.[1]

Recent studies confirm that greater levels of lipoprotein(a) increase the risk and occurrence of CAD, stroke, and the clogging (stenosis) of coronary bypass grafts. So, why does the body make lipoprotein(a) in the first place?

> LDL + apo(a) = lipoprotein(a). Lipoprotein(a) is also referred to as Lp(a).

This Ice Age Genetic Rescue Molecule Solves the Problem and Causes It, Too

Discovered in 1963, lipoprotein(a) is the body's premier artery repairman, traveling to the sites of arterial injuries or lesions. Much like an old hose, the cell membranes become too weak to withstand the constant pressure of the heart pumping blood. The artery ruptures because of a weak collagen structure initiated by deficiencies of vitamin C, lysine, and proline. Lesions appear at the sites where the collagen is incompletely formed. This leaves residues (fragments) of lysine and proline (lysyl residues) at these sites. Complete lysine and proline molecules in the blood prevent the binding of lipoprotein(a) at those sites by actively competing for the space that the residues occupy. Lysine and proline aggressively replace the lysyl residues, forcing them off the lesion site while preventing the attachment of lipoprotein(a) molecules.

Experiments by Dr. Rath confirmed that synthetic lysine was able to bind to lipoprotein(a) and remove it from the artery wall.

Cardiovascular Disease Research Pioneer

Prior to teaming up with Linus Pauling, Dr. Matthias Rath was part of a cardiovascular research team in Germany during the late 1980s. The purpose of that group was to study the plaque from human aortas postmortem (after death). Dr. Rath's team discovered that atherosclerotic plaques were composed primarily of lipoprotein(a), not ordinary LDL cholesterol. After finishing that work, Dr. Rath became a research member of the Linus Pauling Institute of Science and Medicine. There he worked on experiments to examine the relationship between lipoprotein(a) and vitamin C. Those experiments concluded that low intake of vitamin C raised levels of lipoprotein(a) in the blood of test animals compared to controls. Rath and Pauling hypothesized that increased lipoprotein(a) works as a surrogate for vitamin C and hardens blood vessels. Dr. Rath appropriately refers to plaques anchored with lipoprotein(a) as "nature's plaster casts."

Lipoprotein(a) Causes Plaque Deposits and Atherosclerosis

Chronic vitamin C deficiency, or what we call subclinical scurvy syndrome (SSS), causes arteries to become weak throughout the entire cardiovascular system. Wherever there is a weak collagen matrix that ruptures, lipoprotein(a) molecules come rushing to the rescue to patch and plug. The lesions cause accumulations of lipoprotein(a) and other fats to form dangerous plaques. These plaques attract minerals, such as calcium, which harden the plaques, creating a condition called atherosclerosis. As lipoprotein(a) accumulates during the ongoing process of repairing lesion after lesion, it becomes the most significant risk factor for heart attacks and strokes.

The higher the lipoprotein(a) levels in the blood, the more risk there is that lipoprotein(a) will be deposited at the sites of lesions.[2] The larger the vessel wall lesion, the more lipoprotein(a) is deposited. Lipoprotein(a) is one of the largest particles found circulating in the blood and its molecules easily stick together, forming a glob. Once attached to an artery wall, these globs of molecules capture other fat globules in the blood, such as LDL cholesterol, VLDL (very low density lipoprotein) cholesterol, and triglycerides.[3] The fat globules age and cause the immune system response that contributes to the formation of arterial plaque.

Lipoprotein(a) also stimulates the growth of dangerous smooth muscle cells within the artery wall. Lysine and proline competitively inhibit the attachment of lipoprotein(a) to the collagen matrix in the artery wall, enabling the release of lipoprotein(a) and other lipoproteins. Vitamin B_3 (in the form of nicotinic acid—not the niacinamide form) and vitamin C can lower lipoprotein(a).

Doctors Ignore Lipoprotein(a)

Many medical professionals, health practitioners, and experts have mistakenly suggested that we do not bother with lipoprotein(a) since it cannot be controlled. They have not read the research and are unaware that it is a controllable factor in blood.

The Pauling/Rath Inventions and Patents

The ingeniously simple concept behind the therapy of these two geniuses was to significantly increase the intake of the amino acid lysine to nullify the powerful and aggressive binding effect of lipoprotein(a) to artery walls. Their later experiments demonstrated that lysine, along with vitamin C, other amino acids, and antioxidants,

taken regularly in oral amounts far in excess of the established requirements for prevention, were able to inhibit or prevent the attachment
of lipoprotein(a) to artery walls.

When Pauling and Rath submitted laboratory evidence that
clogged arteries could be opened *in vivo* (in living humans), they were
awarded the first two U.S. patents for reversing heart disease without
surgery in 1993 and 1994. Their first patent in 1993 was awarded for
the cleansing and removal of atherosclerotic plaque from human
organs during transplant surgery. The invention consisted of dipping
plaque-coated human organs into a vitamin C and lysine solution. The
plaque on the surface of the organ was melted away by the solution.

According to the second United States patent issued to Pauling and
Rath in 1994, when ample amounts of the amino acids lysine and proline are combined with vitamin C, vitamin E, vitamin A, co-enzyme
Q10, and other antioxidants, they inhibit the binding activity of
lipoprotein(a) to exposed lysine and proline residues. Simply put, these
bionutrients stop plaque from forming and building up on artery walls.
According to Pauling, "large megadoses of Lp(a) binding inhibitors
taken orally, well beyond what we normally consume, raise blood concentrations to therapeutic levels. At these levels, apparently achievable
in most people, the Lp(a) binding inhibitors will prevent and may even
dissolve existing atherosclerotic plaque buildups."

He further commented in the August 1994 issue of the *Journal of
Orthomolecular Nutrition*, "Knowing that lysyl residues are what cause
lipoprotein(a) to get stuck to the wall of the artery and form atherosclerotic plaques, any physical chemist would say at once that the thing
to do is to prevent that by putting the amino acid lysine in the blood
to a greater extent than is normally found. You need lysine to be alive,
it is essential: you have to get about 1 gram a day to keep in protein
balance, but you can take lysine, pure lysine, a perfectly nontoxic substance in foods, as pills, which puts extra lysine molecules in the blood.
They enter into competition with the lysyl residue on the walls of
arteries and accordingly work to prevent lipoprotein(a) from being

deposited, or even will work to pull it loose and destroy atherosclerotic plaques."

Homocysteine and Cardio Destruction

Homocysteine is the quiet cardiovascular killer that has been investigated, examined, and studied for more than twenty years. Currently considered a primary independent risk factor for heart disease, homocysteine, a nonessential amino acid derived from the essential amino acid methionine, builds up swiftly and remains elevated in the blood for years, destroying our arterial linings until the "unthinkable" happens. A deficiency of specific B vitamins is the culprit clearly linked to high homocysteine levels in the blood that damages our arteries. With sufficient folic acid, vitamin B_6 and B_{12}, all easily obtained and ridiculously inexpensive, homocysteine is effortlessly and quickly controlled.

Kilmer S. McCully, M.D.: The Homocysteine Pioneer

In 1969, Kilmer S. McCully, M.D., a young, accomplished molecular biology and genetics researcher at Harvard Medical School, studied the effects of a virtually unknown nonessential amino acid called homocysteine. Little was known about the metabolic role of homocysteine during the early years of Dr. McCully's research.

He continued his homocysteine research at Harvard until 1979, when the head of the department dismissed him, believing that Dr. McCully's years of dedicated research failed to conclusively prove his homocysteine theory of heart disease. His scientific "covered wagon" was unsuccessfully drawn across the medical community terrain for scores of years while his startling research and conclusions were almost totally ignored and dismissed by the medical community as inconclusive and having little medical or scientific merit. His life's work moved forward for more than ten more years and now indisputably proves that homocysteine is a primary independent risk factor for developing heart disease and is of significant clinical importance. Validated, accepted, and employed in the medical, scientific, and lay communities worldwide, it is fast becoming an integral part of cardiovascular diagnostics.

Great News for You

The practical applications of Dr. McCully's theories and findings save and prolong thousands of lives each year. They ensure better health and longer lives for countless more of us than previously possible. His conclusions finally clarify why many aspects of cardiovascular disease are unexplainable. Current cholesterol and fat theories have been incorrectly instilled into the philosophy and practice of the medical community. Scientific experts, medical researchers, and the National Cholesterol Education Program have also misguided the public consciousness for many years.

Excess Homocysteine Increases Your Risk of Cardiovascular Disease

Conclusive and convincing scientific evidence validates homocysteine as a dangerous independent risk and causative factor in the development and progression of cardiovascular disease and cardiovascular accidents. One supportive study in the *Archives of Internal Medicine* (1998) pointed out that in 21,500 men between the ages of thirty-five and sixty-four, those who suffered a heart attack had significantly higher homocysteine levels than those who did not.[4] The study further revealed that subjects with the highest homocysteine levels had a risk factor three to four times greater than those whose levels were lowest.

Another study, reported in the *New England Journal of Medicine* by Dr. Jacob Selhub, examined the relationship of homocysteine levels and carotid artery stenosis in one thousand elderly people, determining that people with the highest levels of homocysteine had double the risk of carotid artery stenosis. Those with the most carotid artery stenosis had the lowest levels of folic acid and B_6.[5] Finally, the Harvard-based Physicians Health Study arrived at fundamentally the same conclusion. Using fifteen thousand male physicians, forty to eighty-four years old for up to five years, it was observed that men with the highest homocysteine levels had about three times the risk of carotid artery stenosis as those with the lowest levels. And it was stated that because high levels of homocysteine can often easily be treated with vitamin supplements, this might be an independent, modifiable risk factor.

Homocysteine Rising

Homocysteine levels in the blood become elevated in three basic ways.

1. DNA strands (strands of our molecular blueprint molecules) are responsible for forming and breaking down homocysteine. Genetic defects in strands that are improperly repaired block the metabolic pathways that reconvert or break down homocysteine.
2. Methionine (an essential amino acid found in all dietary proteins) that is converted in the body to homocysteine is present at much higher levels in animal protein foods than in diets comprised primarily of plant proteins. Meat is the richest source of methionine. This higher concentration dramatically escalates both the potential and the likely amount of homocysteine that can be produced, causing homocysteine levels to become elevated.
3. Deficiencies of folic acid, B_6, and B_{12}, essential B vitamins required to reconvert homocysteine back to methionine or eliminate it from the body, prevent that conversion. This

chronically leaves homocysteine in the blood at hazardously high and rising levels.

According to Dr. McCully, high homocysteine levels in the blood are caused primarily by nutritional deficiencies of folic acid, B_6, and B_{12}, plus genetic, toxic, hormonal, and aging factors. The presence or absence of these factors within us is the key to the proper formation and metabolic activity of the three enzymes (cysthathione b-synthase, methylenetetrahydrofolate reductase, and methyl transferase) considered vital in breaking down homocysteine. Dietary factors contributing to the total content of methionine and the levels of folic acid, B_6, and B_{12} circulating in the blood predominantly determine whether or not homocysteine levels will elevate.

Homocysteine can only be formed from methionine. Dr. McCully points out that plant proteins contain significantly less methionine than animal proteins, strongly suggesting that we can limit the body's potential to form excess harmful homocysteine from methionine by controlling the quantity of animal protein consumed in the diet. It also explains why populations that consume a plant-based diet are relatively protected against arteriosclerosis and atherosclerosis. In contrast, populations such as ours, that consume a diet rich in meat and dairy products, are afforded minimal protection and are subject to high risk. Lower dietary levels of methionine generate lower levels of homocysteine, requiring less metabolic work, less folic acid, B_6, and B_{12} to convert homocysteine back to methionine or into cysthathionine. When we consume animal-based diets rich in red meat, pork, poultry, and dairy, the need for folic acid, B_6, and B_{12} increases dramatically to accomplish this task.

Smoking is a primary toxic factor that causes homocysteine to rise. Imbalances of our thyroid hormones and lower postmenopausal hormone levels allow homocysteine to increase in the blood, too. Finally, the normal aging process itself pushes homocysteine up beyond healthy levels.

Homocysteine Thiolactone: An Artery Enemy

Homocysteine undergoes a metabolic change that converts it to an extremely destructive artery enemy. That substance is called homocysteine thiolactone. It is a highly reactive and extremely dangerous form of homocysteine that attacks and destroys protein molecules in the artery linings. It makes them weak and susceptible to damage, initiating the Cardiovascular Metabolic Repair Response.

The Hajar study presented in the *Journal of Clinical Investigation* (1993) suggested that homocysteine circulating in the blood directly promotes blood clotting and initiates debilitating strokes and heart attacks. How? It does this by reducing the number of available binding sites for the natural anticlotting factor of tissue plasminogen (t-PA). This reduction in the number of t-PA binding sites triggers more clots to form that block the flow of blood.

Homocysteine thiolactone is understood to aggregate (clot) low-density lipoprotein cholesterol, also known as the "bad cholesterol." These LDL–homocysteine aggregates (clumps) are pulled on to the artery wall by white blood cells called macrophages sent by the immune system. Foam cells are formed and lay the foundation for plaques that initiate atherosclerosis on arterial walls. These foam cells also break down the LDL–homocysteine aggregates and release destructive oxidized fats and cholesterol into developing plaques. Homocysteine thiolactone is also released into other surrounding cells of the arterial wall, negatively affecting the way these cells handle and process oxygen. Consequently, highly reactive oxygen-free radicals form and accumulate in cells that line the arterial wall. This encourages the formation of life-threatening blood clots, unwanted arterial muscle cells, and other hard, fibrous tissues that severely reduce the elasticity and flexibility of the artery. Stiffer and more rigid than before, those arteries are vulnerable to cracking or rupturing readily, much like an old rubber hose.

Banish Homocysteine with Simple B Vitamins

Blood homocysteine levels are controlled by a combination of nutritional and genetic factors, among which is the enzyme methylenetetrahydrofolate reductase (MTHFR). A defective variation of this enzyme is unmistakably associated with elevated homocysteine. Increased blood plasma levels of homocysteine are directly linked to a genetic inheritance of this defective enzyme. In 1996, researchers at the Department of Genetics at Trinity College in Dublin, Ireland, reported in *Circulation* that the presence of the defective MTHFR enzyme apparently amplified the risk of premature coronary artery disease. They concluded that genetically correct MTHFR, which effectively controls homocysteine concentrations in the blood, is totally dependent on folic acid. Supplementation may reduce the risk.[6]

Each year nearly fifteen million people die from various cardiovascular diseases, particularly from heart attacks and strokes. Some form of heart disease causes 50 percent of all deaths in the United States. In 1995, approximately 455,000 men and 505,000 women died from cardiovascular disease. The value of folic acid, B_6, and B_{12} vitamins for controlling and reducing homocysteine in the blood cannot be overstated. The 1998 Rimm-Willet study in the *Journal of the American Medical Association* established the relationship and significance of folate and vitamin B_6 in preventing cardiovascular disease.[7] The earlier Boushey study in the *Journal of the American Medical Association* (1995) suggested that we could prevent 13,500 to 50,000 deaths from cardiovascular diseases by including about twenty-five cents' worth of B vitamins in the daily diet.[8]

Convincing scientific information suggests that lowering the risk of heart disease, sudden death, and early mortality can be accomplished by supplementing with folic acid. A revealing study in *The Lancet* (1998) examined thirty-eight patients with a combination of progressive atherosclerosis of their carotid arteries and high homocysteine levels.

During an eighteen-month trial period the group was given supplemental folic acid, B_6, and B_{12}. The promising result: Arterial lesions stopped progressing and regressed slightly, suggesting that similar results could be achieved in larger population studies.

Another eye-opening study presented in *Journal of the American Medical Association* (1996) stated that a minimum of 13,500 deaths from coronary artery disease could be prevented each year by simply increasing the intake of folic acid to lower homocysteine levels in the blood. Furthermore, a 1998 study published in the *Annals of Epidemiology* took a close look at the relationship of folate and coronary heart disease risk. The results put forth the hypothesis that risk factors for heart disease due to a lack of folic acid were age related and that risk increased with age. There's no doubt that we can normalize homocysteine with B vitamins.

Push Back the Enemy Naturally: Eat Beets

Three significant metabolic processes occur within the body that control how much homocysteine circulates in our blood.

Methylation: This complicated metabolic process beneficially
   modifies and protects the basic structure of DNA, our
   genetic blueprint molecules, by attaching special methyl
   molecules to molecules of DNA.

Remethylation: A reversible biochemical process that uses
   folic acid and vitamin B_{12} to reconvert homocysteine back
   into the harmless essential amino acid methionine.

Transsulfuration: An irreversible process that teams up
   vitamin B_6 with the enzyme cysthathionine b-synthase to
   convert homocysteine to cysthathionine and then to cystine,
   a harmless nonessential amino acid that is excreted in the
   urine.

Research points out that the lowest levels of homocysteine in the blood are associated with the lowest risk of cardiovascular disease. Conversely, the highest levels of homocysteine are associated with the highest risk. By constantly changing homocysteine back to methionine or converting it to harmless cysteine and clearing it from the blood, we dramatically reduce the cardiovascular risk and cardio destruction that too much homocysteine can cause.

Beets are a rich source of choline and betaine. Choline is a precursor to betaine (not to be confused with betaine hydrochloride—stomach acid). Betaine is also called trimethylglycine (TMG), a very active methyl donor that will assist in converting homocysteine back to methionine, while protecting the DNA in our cells.

Elevated Homocysteine and Early Death

Current bionutritional research suggests that 6 micromoles of homocysteine per liter in the blood represents low to no risk of cardiovascular disease, while 10 micromoles per liter indicate an increased risk. Thirteen micromoles per liter are considered very dangerous. When homocysteine levels increase far above 13, a heart attack or stroke is just waiting to happen. Sufficient supplementation with folic acid, B_6, and B_{12}, along with a reduction of methionine-rich animal protein food should be incorporated into the diet. Follow-up testing should be performed periodically to monitor homocysteine levels and adjust vitamin and dietary therapy.

Blood Sugar Disorders and Syndrome X

At the center of all dysglycemias (blood sugar disorders) lie insulin and glucose.

Insulin: Dysglycemia Kingpin

Insulin is a metabolic friend and foe. It is a hormone produced by the islets of Langerhans, a "hormone factory" in your pancreas. It controls and regulates blood sugar levels and the storage of glycogen, another form of glucose that is stored in the muscles and liver. Glycogen can immediately be converted back to glucose for energy. When there is excess glycogen in the liver it is converted to triglycerides, which move into the blood and get stored as adipose tissue—fat.

Insulin at Work in the Body

When glucose (blood sugar) rises as a result of the ingestion of food, your pancreas releases insulin. Your cells receive a signal to take in the glucose. It is then metabolized for energy or easily stored in a water-based form called glycogen. After a while, your blood sugar levels begin to drop, because the body is using up glucose for energy. When blood sugar levels fall too low, the pancreas pumps out the hormone glucagon to convert glycogen stored in muscles back to glucose. Then insulin is released again to assist glucose metabolism. In many people, the muscles miss the signal and glucose does not get taken up into the cells. This is called insulin resistance. With glucose levels still high, your pancreas continues to produce more insulin. This results in excessively high levels of insulin circulating in the blood.

Why is this bad? Excess insulin will raise triglycerides and lower HDL cholesterol. But it will not raise LDL cholesterol. Excess triglycerides will circulate in the blood. The longer they swim around, the more likely they are to become victims of free radical damage. Once damaged, triglycerides will stick more readily to artery walls. Lower HDL cholesterol levels means less LDL cholesterol returning to the liver for breakdown and excretion. It also means that the LDL/HDL cholesterol ratio will be higher, suggesting more cardiovascular risk.

Although insulin does not increase the level of LDL cholesterol, it causes the worst damage by significantly affecting the size of LDL cholesterol particles. Studies published in the *Journal of Clinical Investigation* (1993), conducted by expert researcher Dr. Gerald Reaven and colleagues, tells us that the number of smaller-diameter, highly atherogenic (producing atherosclerotic plaques) LDL cholesterol particles increases dramatically with the degree of insulin resistance. Finally, excess unmetabolized glucose will attach to proteins in the artery walls, form AGES (Advanced Glycation/Glycosylation End Substances), and damage the walls.

Too Much of a Good Thing Is Dangerous: Insulin Destroys Arteries

The most important role of insulin is to transport glucose to receptor sites on cell membranes, so that glucose can be metabolized for energy within the cell. Excess insulin that circulates in the blood for too long erodes and tears down arterial linings, initiating the CMRR process. From infancy through adulthood, many people develop resistance to the proper function of insulin and efficient glucose uptake.

In 1997, a study by O. Lindberg at the University of Helsinki, Finland, questioned whether insulin was an independent risk factor for cardiovascular disease. The study examined fasting plasma insulin with CVD and the ability to use insulin as a CVD predictor. The results were quite interesting. People with CVD generally had higher fasting insulin levels than those without CVD. Heart failure and hypertension were associated with 30 to 80 percent elevations in insulin in all age groups, except the oldest.[9] Lindberg concluded that insulin, though a strong contributor to CVD, was not clearly an independent risk factor. We disagree. Lindberg's findings clearly indicate that insulin is a very reactive and dangerous contributor to heart disease. While the technical criteria for classifying insulin as an independent risk factor may not have been met, it does, independently of other risk factors, cause sufficient cardiovascular damage to consider it an independent risk factor.

Glucose: The Body's Primary Energy Source

Technically, glucose is what scientists call a monosaccharide, a simple sugar. In fact, it is the simplest of sugars and serves as the body's primary dietary source of metabolic cellular energy. Glucose in the body is derived from food, primarily dietary sugars and carbohydrates. It can also be produced from nonsugar or noncarbohydrate sources, such as the amino acids in proteins and glycerol from the breakdown of fats (triglyceride) in fat cells, whenever necessary. This glucose-generating process is called gluconeogenesis. Glucose, via a series of chemical steps called a metabolic pathway, is converted into ATP (adenosine triphosphate), the body's primary energy molecule. It is escorted by insulin into special receptors located on the surface of fat and muscle cells so that it can be converted into energy.

The Sugar-Insulin Metabolic Cycle

Now let's consider the sugar-insulin metabolic cycle. When we consume food, the sugar and carbohydrate portions of it are converted to glucose. Ideally, your pancreas will secrete an appropriate amount of insulin to escort glucose to special spots on cell membranes, called receptor sites, where the glucose can enter the cells. If there are too few receptor sites or if there is resistance to glucose entry, then insulin resistance (turning away insulin) and glucose resistance occur. This leaves an excess of insulin and glucose circulating in the blood. Both are cardioirritants. Normally, glucose concentration in the blood under average fasting conditions is approximately 70 to 90 milligrams per 100 milliliters of blood. When we consume food, it is broken down into its various components: fats, proteins, and carbohydrates. When sugar/carbohydrate is eaten, blood sugar levels rise typically to 90 to 140 milligrams per 100 milliliters of blood, creating a condition called hyperglycemia. Above 140, the renal threshold (the maximum level the kidneys can hold) is reached. At 140 to 170, the kidneys spill excess glucose into the urine. When glucose is below fasting level, less than 70, hypoglycemia occurs.

Glucose Is Controlled by Three Hormones

During a carbohydrate-rich meal we become hyperglycemic, and insulin escorts glucose into cells to be metabolized, or lowers glucose levels by increasing glucose conversion to glycogen, thus normalizing blood sugar. Excess insulin production to overcompensate for too much glucose typically pushes blood sugar down too low, causing temporary hypoglycemia, which triggers glucagon and adrenalin to again convert glucose to glycogen. Conversely, glucagon from the pancreas and adrenalin from the adrenal glands increase the rate of glycogen breakdown and increase blood glucose levels when energy is needed.

Priming the Glucagon Gun

When the body pumps up this anti-fat storage hormone to stimulate and accelerate the conversion of glycogen in the liver into glucose on demand for energy, insulin levels are reduced. Glucagon prevents the conversion of stored glycogen into triglycerides, which then converts to body fat. Because glucagon is an insulin antagonist and opposes the production of insulin, a fat-storage hormone, it also brings stored fats back into the blood to be metabolized. One of the simplest ways to increase glucagon levels in the blood and consequently prevent the storage of fat is to exercise regularly, which will require energy in the form of glucose that will be metabolized rather than ultimately stored as body fat.

Tips for Preventing the "Spike": Balancing Blood Sugar Naturally

To prevent the sudden "spikes" (sharp rises) and dips in blood sugar levels that result from a diet comprised of simple sugars and carbohydrates, replace them with complex carbohydrates, such as whole wheat breads and pasta; brown rice; whole grains, such as quinoa, amaranth, spelt, teff and millet; legumes; vegetables; and soy foods.

- Eat small, frequent meals.
- Eat low–glycemic index foods.
- Take targeted supplements and herbs.
- Drink lots of quality water.
- Exercise regularly.

The Glycemic Index

The *glycemic index* is a term used to illustrate the body's blood glucose response to the consumption of a specific food. Using a measured quantity of glucose to raise blood sugar to a specified level, the index shows how equal quantities of other foods raise blood sugar by comparison to glucose. Values are based on single foods eaten alone.

Foods with a high value raise blood sugar rapidly and spike insulin levels in the blood. Continued spiking of blood sugar overstimulates and stresses the pancreas, causing too much insulin to be produced. This overproduction of insulin ultimately drives blood sugar levels down too low, creating a need for more blood sugar. This initiates a hyperglycemic (high blood sugar) and hypoglycemic (low blood sugar) yo-yo response that causes fatigue and weakness and turns on the appetite/hunger response at the hypoglycemic valley of the blood sugar curve. Be aware that refined carbohydrates (white sugars and flours) easily spike insulin levels, causing a vicious cycle of highs and lows in your energy level and the appetite/hunger response. Imbalances in sugar metabolism set the stage for a variety of health problems, among them insulin resistance, Syndrome X, and worst of all, diabetes.

Do You Have Syndrome X?

Either as a result of genetic defects or the long-term abuse of blood sugar metabolism by diets high in simple sugars and refined carbohydrates, we develop resistance to the proper function of insulin and the efficient uptake and metabolism of glucose. Under normal blood sugar/insulin production conditions, glucose is efficiently cleared from the blood and glucose levels return to normal. Insulin resistance means that body tissues do not respond normally to insulin and an excessive amount is needed to bring blood glucose back into balance. This is caused in part by a reduced number of special cells, called target cells, which have insulin receptors that can accept glucose. According to a functional medicine update published last year in *Physiological Reviews*, insulin resistance, a major part of Syndrome X, is reported to affect an estimated 25 percent of adults in the United States.[10] Insulin resistance is predominant in people who have diabetes, who have high blood pressure, or are obese. Heredity is also an influencing factor.

The Damaging Effects of Insulin Resistance

There are many harmful aspects of insulin resistance, including:

- Elevated blood pressure
- Reduced removal of LDL cholesterol
- Deposition of LDL cholesterol
- Hyperinsulinemia (chronically high insulin levels)
- High blood glucose levels
- Elevated triglycerides and VLDL cholesterol
- Lowered HDL cholesterol levels

This group of conditions is known collectively as Syndrome X, which increases the risk of coronary artery disease, diabetes, and obesity. It's a vicious cycle. Obesity, a result of insulin resistance, causes elevated insulin and insulin resistance all over again.

Your diet is key to whether you have or will develop insulin resistance.

Factors That Increase Your Chances of Developing Insulin Resistance

Contributing factors toward developing insulin resistance include:

1. A diet high in sugar and refined carbohydrates has a high glycemic index and will raise your insulin levels rapidly because glucose from simple sugars and refined carbohydrates enter the blood fast.

2. A high ratio of omega-6 EFAs (essential fatty acid) to omega-3 EFAs, or EFA deficiency will cause you to have insulin resistance. Cell membranes that contain the most unsaturated fatty acids become the most fluid and have the most insulin receptors. This increases insulin sensitivity and the amount of glucose that gets taken up by the cells.[11]

3. High amounts of trans-fatty acids (TFAs) get in the way of fatty acid metabolism. They crowd out EFAs from cell membranes and prevent omega-3 fatty acids like alpha-linolenic acid from converting to DA, the most unsaturated and fluid fatty acid.

Test Yourself for Insulin Resistance

Get out the scale and tape measure! Obesity is a contributing factor to the development of insulin resistance. A waist-to-hip ratio greater than 1 for men and greater than .88 for women is a good predictor of heart disease. To measure and calculate the ratio, simply take measurements of your waist and hips and divide the waist measurement by the hip measurement to obtain the ratio.

Get blood tests that measure the levels of glucose and lipids in the blood. Insulin resistance (hyperinsulinemia) raises triglycerides and lowers HDL. Impaired glucose tolerance (fasting glucose 111 to 125 milligrams per 100 milliliters of blood) often indicates insulin resistance, according to the 1997 criteria published by the American Diabetes Association. Elevated fasting levels of insulin and/or elevated levels two hours after a glucose challenge test indicates an increased secretion of insulin indicative of insulin resistance.

Diabetes: The Silent Epidemic

The Bubonic Plague . . . the Black Death . . . and diabetes? Most of us imagine an epidemic as some virtually incurable, horrible disease, ravaging some faraway place. Surprisingly, diabetes spearheads a silent epidemic that causes needless suffering for nearly twenty million Americans, and this number is rapidly on the rise. In fact, diabetes is the fourth leading cause of death in the United States and the foremost cause of cardiovascular disease, kidney disease, and blindness. The devastating dangers of diabetes have endured lengthy discussion.

Professor John Yudkin's 1972 classic book, *Sweet and Dangerous*, clearly spelled out the horrifying health hazards of sugar, insulin imbalance, and diabetes. Robert Atkins, M.D., a New York physician, has been discussing the dangers of sugar and refined carbohydrates for more than twenty-five years. The long-term damage of this dreaded disease occurs when complications arise, according to a report published by Sabinsa Corporation entitled "Diabetes—Its Etiology and Control with Ayurvedic Herbs." As researchers and the American Diabetic Association continue the search for a cure, they remain somewhat unaware or naive to the knowledge that diabetes responds exceptionally well to natural treatments.

Diabetes Rising: Understanding the Dilemma

The ancient Sanskrit referred to diabetes as *madhumeha* (honey urine) because of the sweet smell and taste imparted to the urine of diabetics. Diabetes is a chronic disorder distinguished by high blood sugar; abnormal carbohydrate, fat, and protein metabolism; insufficient production and/or inefficient usage of insulin to regulate blood sugar; and insulin resistance. When insulin does not fit into special receptors that unlock the gateway allowing glucose to enter the cells, insulin resistance results. Muscles become starved of glucose and excessive fat metabolism produces deleterious by-products, such as ketones, that enter the blood.

The classic symptoms of diabetes, including frequent urination, excessive thirst, and excessive appetite, can lead to chronic brain fog, faintness, and coma. Obesity is an additional independent factor triggering diabetes, since overweight people appear to have fewer insulin receptor sites than those of normal weight. Lack of exercise and excess stress also contribute to the onset of diabetes.

Diabetes 1, 2, 3

There are three types of diabetes:

1. **IDDM-I, Type I:** Insulin-dependent diabetes mellitus (IDDM) occurs most often in young children and adolescents. Type I affects 10 percent of diabetics. This commonly results from early injury to insulin-producing beta cells in the pancreas as an outcome of a faulty autoimmune response or poor tissue-regenerating capacity. In Type I diabetics, beta cells don't produce any insulin at all.

2. **NIDDM-II, Type II:** Noninsulin-dependent diabetes mellitus (NIDDM) usually occurs after age forty. Type II, reported to affect 90 percent of diabetics, most often develops when the pancreas does not secrete enough insulin to properly clear glucose from blood. In other diabetics, the

beta cells overproduce insulin because of insulin resistance. Cells become resistant to insulin, preventing the proper entry of glucose. Faulty beta cells in the pancreas or an insufficient number of them are the culprits. Research suggests that diets containing excess refined carbohydrates also play a strong role in initiating Type II diabetes.

3. **Gestational diabetes:** This type of diabetes occurs in about 5 percent of pregnancies and is usually temporary, disappearing soon after childbirth. Gestational diabetes that does not resolve and disappear within a short while after childbirth suggests a more complex blood sugar problem, a cardiovascular problem, or both.

Allopathic Medical Treatment: A Failure in Disguise

In a conversation with Steve French, Senior Vice President at the Natural Marketing Institute of Telford, Pennsylvania, we learned that approximately nineteen to twenty-one million people are now actively managing diabetes. Unfortunately, allopathic (conventional) medical treatment for diabetes remains merely a finger in the dike. Its primary goal is to treat symptoms and maintain normal blood sugar levels by attempting to increase insulin sensitivity with regular doses of oral or injectable insulin ordered by the doctor. It does not address cardiovascular damage, diabetic neuropathy (nerve damage), kidney damage, and other problems that usually develop as complications of the disease. When these complications arise, the treatment of choice is to prescribe more drugs to suppress the growing symptoms, while continuing to ignore the primary causes.

Good Glycemic Index Gobbling

The key to balanced blood sugar is the consumption of low–glycemic index foods that do not spike insulin. Far and away, soy is the diabetic's best friend. And in this exploding category there are numerous choices. Items like sugar-free soy shakes and meal replacement bars, and foods such as tofu, textured vegetable protein (TVP), and soynut butter are excellent choices. Refer to the glycemic index in part VII.

Putting It All Together

Diabetes, dysglycemia, insulin resistance, and Syndrome X are dangerous dietary disorders that are rapidly rising to epidemic levels. Their occurrence and long-term systemic damage can be successfully controlled or eliminated with the use of targeted nutritional supplements, healthy natural foods, natural therapies, and exercise.

Arterial Inflammation

Inflammation is the pain, heat, redness, swelling, and loss of function we experience, that results from the body's localized protective response to injury or destruction of tissues. The inflammation attempts to wall off, destroy, and dilute the injurious agent and the injured tissue. The inflammatory response dilates the arterioles (small arteries), capillaries, and venules (small veins), increasing their permeability. This allows the elimination of fluids and the arrival of leukocytes (white blood cells) at the injury site.

Inflammation can arise silently anywhere in the body, especially in the artery wall. The latest hypothesis about the cause of heart disease is pointed at the body's own defenses—the immune system and the mechanism by which it causes the inflammation. This, too, is cause and effect. The injury, as previously explained (caused by free radicals, homoscyteine thiolactone, glucose, oxidized LDL cholesterol, and bacteria attacking artery linings), is the cause. And the inflammation, along with the biochemical and physiological response it brings, is the effect.

According to an expert on the subject of arterial inflammation, Aftab Ahmed, Ph.D., Director of Research and Development and

Business Development at Marlyn Nutriceuticals, Scottsdale, Arizona, "the turncoat mechanism responsible for the onset of many chronic diseases is inflammation. An increasing amount of data suggests that inflammation may well be at the core of coronary artery disease (CAD) as well."[12]

Dr. Ahmed is not alone in his scientific thinking. A 1999 paper by biomedical researcher R. Ross, published in the *New England Journal of Medicine*, established that atherosclerosis is an inflammatory process.[13] Heart attacks are believed to result from long-term cycles of injury, inflammation, repair, and re-injury inside blood vessels, causing the deposition and buildup of repair molecules such as lipoprotein(a), cholesterol, and platelets.[14]

That Greasy Buildup

The first sign of impending plaque buildup inside the artery is systemic inflammation caused by an irritation or injury. This event on the artery wall can be initiated by factors like oxidized cholesterol, free radicals, homocysteine, high blood pressure, and smoking. As previously mentioned, repeated injuries to endothelial cells that make up the endothelium cause the formation of cell adhesion molecules (CAMs).

These CAMs, in turn, start a healing/repair process by placing a biochemical ID tag on the cell. This tag identifies the enemy, and a signal for help is sent. In the blood vessel network, CAMs summon white blood cells called monocytes from the immune system. They attach to the blood vessel lining and squeeze among the endothelial cells. This causes inflammation in the underlying tissue. The monocytes are transformed into macrophages, the "garbage cleaner" cells of the immune system.

CAMs and macrophages collect cholesterol, lipoprotein(a), and platelets that travel to the injury site to repair the damage. Then, a protein coating called a fibrous cap forms over the developing plaque. The plaques continue to mature by collecting lipoprotein(a), LDL cholesterol, oxidized LDL cholesterol, triglycerides, other fats, and calcium. These deposits begin to harden and calcify, becoming more stiff and inflexible as they grow. The mature and fully developed plaques stabilize, calcify, harden, remain fixed, and rarely rupture. Eventually, they can occupy 70 percent or more of the potential blood volume of the artery, severely restricting blood flow and causing angina. In the case of a complete blockage, they initiate a debilitating or potentially fatal stroke or heart attack.

Watch Out for the Little Guys

Younger, less developed plaques are softer and have a thinner fibrous cap. They occupy only 30 to 40 percent of blood vessel volume but are significantly more volatile. These extremely dangerous little plaques, unlike their much larger, harder, artery-choking counterparts, cause no outward or measurable symptoms because blood vessel walls expand in response to their growth, and the blockages cannot be detected. Thus, they go unnoticed in angiograms.

As with older, larger plaques, the immune response continues to attract monocytes from the immune system, which become macrophages that soak up cholesterol, lipoprotein(a), and platelets. These cells also become bloated, and foam cells form. The macrophages then burst and die. Their cell sap (contents) exits under the fibrous cap into the bulk of the plaque. This cellular garbage is rich in proteins that destroy and destabilize the cap. Macrophages also release tissue factor, which increases the potential of blood to clot. This destabilized plaque is vulnerable to a localized increase in blood pressure that triggers the plaque to burst. Finally, these younger plaques become fatigued and rupture, forming sudden massive clots that cause a heart attack or stroke. We have identified the problem. What, then, is the marker used to measure this inflammation indicative of atherosclerosis?

C-Reactive Protein: A Better Marker of Heart Disease than Cholesterol

C-reactive protein (CRP) is a biochemical inflammation marker that elevates when systemic inflammation is present. According to Dr. Ahmed, "It is an acute-phase protein produced in the liver as a defense mechanism to a wide range of stimuli." C-reactive protein is normally found in low concentration in healthy individuals. It is highly concentrated in those with inflammation, bacterial or viral infections, cellular injuries, and inflammatory diseases, such as rheumatoid arthritis. Increasingly, it is being chosen as a diagnostic test for the prediction of disease in healthy people, especially to predict coronary artery disease (CAD).

Recent studies by Paul M. Ridker, M.D., Charles H. Hennekens, M.D., and research colleagues have demonstrated clearly that measurement of existing levels of CRP in the blood is perhaps the most reliable predictor of CAD. Dr. Ridker is the focal point and primary researcher in landmark studies about inflammation, CRP, and heart disease. His latest study was published in the *New England Journal of Medicine* (March 2000). It examined and evaluated C-reactive protein along with eleven other biomarkers of inflammation, such as total cholesterol, homocysteine, interleukin-6, low-density lipoprotein, CAMs, and others, as a tool for predicting heart disease in women. Earlier studies were conducted on men and women, although this study was not gender sensitive.[15]

In conjunction with the findings of their earlier research, Drs. Ridker and Hennekens concluded that chronic inflammation plays a strong role in the onset and development of CAD, and that hs-CRP (highly sensitive C-reactive protein) was the strongest predictor of cardiovascular events of the twelve biomarkers studied.[16] The studies concluded that an elevated level of CRP is a strong warning signal that a negative cardiac event is impending. This is in no way the only marker to be considered or used to make an evaluation. Dr. Ridker continues to study the role of inflammation and C-reactive protein in the onset and development of CAD. Another significant finding resulted from this study. Fifty percent of all heart attacks occur in people whose plasma lipid levels are normal![17]

A logical question to ask is: what therapy or therapies lend themselves to the reduction or elimination of inflammation within the system? Dr. Ahmed tells us that systemic and digestive enzymes, such as trypsin, papain, and bromelain, have clearly demonstrated their ability to reduce chronic systemic inflammation.[18]

The Clotting Factors

In 1863, Joseph Lister, surgeon to Queen Victoria and the founder of antiseptic surgery, conducted the first studies of how the body uses the clotting mechanism as a repair mode.[19]

Fibrinogen: An Independent Risk Factor

Fibrinogen is a component of the blood essential to the clotting process. Many health professionals consider fibrinogen to be a totally harmless protein unless activated by thrombin. But this assumption is not at all true. Fibrinogen is an acute-phase (emergency need) protein made in the liver and is a co-factor for platelet aggregation. It determines the viscosity of blood and stimulates the formation of plaque.

In 1994, Dr. E. Ernst conducted the Northwick Park Heart Study in the United Kingdom. It analyzed 1,510 men, aged forty to sixty-four, for clotting factors including fibrinogen. Dr. Ernst observed the activity of fibrinogen in the blood and concluded it to be an important risk factor for atherosclerosis.[20]

Fibrinogen is an enzyme precursor to fibrin, the major active clotting factor in our blood. In 1996, Dr. G. B. Rosito of the Institute for the Prevention of Cardiovascular Disease at Deaconess Hospital,

Harvard Medical School, Boston, stated in a journal review that fibrinogen had been identified as an independent risk factor for cardiovascular disease that was as powerful a predictor as cholesterol.[21] Any injury that causes a blood vessel to

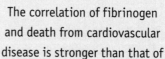

The correlation of fibrinogen and death from cardiovascular disease is stronger than that of cholesterol and CVD.

break sets off a chain of events to repair the rupture. Platelets in the blood immediately change their shape from round to spiny. They migrate to the break in the blood vessel wall, attaching to it and to each other. Von Willebrand factor, a protein made by the artery walls, assists platelets to stick. There they hook up with clotting factors in blood, especially thrombin. When a link of protein in fibrinogen is removed with the aid of thrombin (an enzyme stored in the body as prothrombin), it becomes the active factor fibrin. Fibrin is essentially the glue our blood produces to clot when necessary. Fibers of fibrin form a net that traps more platelets, and so on, plugging the leak.

As molecules of fibrin aggregate (clump together), they rapidly form in a snowball effect, accumulating as a fibrous clump. This is what we call a clot. Under normal conditions, the electrical charge of fibrinogen keeps it from bonding together, whereas an opposite electrical charge, with the aid of thrombin, stimulates fibrin molecules to bind together. Omega-3 fatty acids reduce the production of fibrinogen. Vitamin K, a fat-soluble vitamin, is essential to the formation of prothrombin and other clotting factors. Familiar blood thinners like the prescription drug Coumadin (a type of warfarin also used in rat poison) work by thinning the blood so much that even the slightest rupture would cause an animal to bleed to death.[22]

Clotting however, must be precisely controlled, as there is a fine line between hemorrhaging and clotting. The body makes anticlotting factors to control the reaction time of clotting activity. The most prominent anticlotting factor is Antithrombin III. Heparin is a polysaccharide (complex sugar) found in special mast cells of the immune system and on the surface of endothelial cells lining the artery wall. It works as an anticoagulant by increasing the rate at which anticlotting factors form.

It's important to keep in mind that clots are not permanent appendages. In fact, human genetics has designed them to be broken up when the injury has healed. For that there is fibrinolysis, a metabolic process in which plasmin chops and splits up fibrin, causing it to degrade and dissolve.

Fibrinogen + thrombin
(a proteolytic enzyme)
> fibrin

Plasmin is stored as t-PA (tissue plasminogen activator), a substance that is converted to plasminogen and then to plasmin. But plasmin levels decrease with age, causing blood flow problems. Sluggish blood and narrowing of arterial deposits increase the risk of clotting. In contrast, fibrinogen levels, along with their increased fibrin production, rise with age. Levels of clotting factors escalate and clot-busting factors diminish. This increases the risk of angina, heart attack, and stroke. Fibrin is also believed to promote the dangerous proliferation of smooth muscle cells that we discussed in chapter 2.

Platelet Aggregation

Studies show that abnormally excessive aggregation of platelets is a serious risk factor for heart disease and strokes. When they clump and stick to the artery wall, platelets produce compounds that accelerate formation of plaques.[23] The stickiness of platelets is affected by the amount of saturated fats, cholesterol, and antioxidant levels in the blood. Healthy, essential omega-3 fats prevent platelet aggregation and the risk of clotting while saturated and trans fats stimulate platelet aggregation. Basic vitamins, such as B_6, inhibit platelet aggregation. This was reported in a 1980 study by Arfenist, Lam, and colleagues.[24]

A more recent study in 1995, in the German journal *Arnzeim Forsch*, supported Lam's earlier findings that simple B_6 could effectively reduce a serious cardiovascular risk factor.[25] New research, revealed by

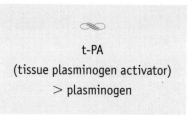

t-PA
(tissue plasminogen activator)
> plasminogen

C. Pace-Asciak in 1995, points to resveratrol, a potent polyphenol in red wine grapes and red wine that exerts powerful antiplatelet activity.[26]

Congenital Defects: Good Genes, Bad Genes

Finally, we must consider how CVD is influenced by factors that present themselves in the womb. During the eighth to tenth weeks after conception, the fetal heart fully develops. By the time the fetal heart is no larger than a peanut, any congenital defects that are programmed to develop in the young heart are already present. Deformities, such as valve damage, holes in muscular tissue separating the chambers, a pinched or narrowed aorta, and blue baby syndrome (when part of the blood that is returning from the body does not pick up oxygen in the lungs because the aorta and pulmonary artery are reversed) are the congenital defects usually seen in developing fetuses and newborns. Each year, about 25,000 babies are born with these defects and about 5,500 infant deaths result from them.

NINE

Nutritional Factors

Just Say No to Sugar, Glucose, and AGES

The significant dangers of sugar and refined carbohydrates were first explained in 1957 by noted English professor John Yudkin. After many epidemiological and clinical studies, he concluded in his 1971 publication *Sugar: Chemical, Biological, and Nutritional Aspects of Sucrose*, that "men who consumed high quantities of sugar had a significantly greater risk of CVD than those who had low intake of sugar."[1] His classic 1972 book, *Sweet and Dangerous*, further discussed the dangerous role of refined sugar in heart disease.

AGES (Advanced Glycation/Glycosylation End Substances): The Glycation Reaction

Glycation is the process whereby excess glucose reacts with "building block" proteins in the body. Certain sugars—glucose (blood sugar), along with ribose and fructose (fruit sugar)—produced from excess dietary sugars and refined carbohydrates, eagerly enter into spontaneous reactions with collagen, the major body protein in connective tissue. These sugars continually attach to proteins in the arterial wall. This accelerates aging by forming free radicals that cause structurally unsound cross-linking of proteins. Cross-linking causes free radicals and DNA to stick together, preventing DNA from making what the body needs. Instead, this produces useless debris. The glycation reaction causes the proteins to stop functioning properly and is responsible for forming brownish fluorescent structures called AGES (Advanced Glycation End Substances).[2] These are proteins damaged by sugar and other complex derivatives of glucose.

AGES damage and destroy arterial linings by changing their physical and chemical characteristics. As a result, the body loses cells and produces waste that clogs and stiffens tissue. The damage that alters these cells makes them susceptible to injury, and the stiffness makes them more resistant to blood flow. Blood pressure increases, which can exacerbate or hasten the rupture of an artery and alter structural integrity. This initiates the Cardiovascular Metabolic Repair Response and accelerates the rate at which we age. The damage caused by sugar is just as serious as the damage that is caused by reactive forms of oxygen. Reducing blood sugar levels will decrease the ability of glucose to latch on to proteins in the artery wall and destroy them.

Excess glycation activity has many negative side effects, such as impaired immunity, damage to proteins that regulate body functions, damage to structural proteins, and the breakdown of metabolic enzymes required for proper metabolism. Reducing glycation activity in the body lowers the risk for three significant age-related diseases: heart disease, cancer, and arthritis. The great danger is that

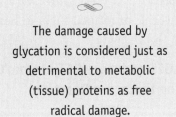

The damage caused by glycation is considered just as detrimental to metabolic (tissue) proteins as free radical damage.

the rate at which these artery-destroying AGES form is directly related to the amount of glucose circulating in the blood and the length of time it circulates.

What does this mean? Diets that are high in simple sugars and refined carbohydrates that rapidly convert to simple sugars create more glycation and more cross-linking damage to cells than diets moderately comprised of refined sugars and carbohydrates. Diabetics, whose sugar levels are typically high, have much more glucose circulating more of the time than nondiabetics. The major point to consider is that this causes damage to collagen throughout the circulatory system, particularly in the coronary arteries of the heart, head, and eyes. This results in injury and repair activity, plaque development, heart attacks, strokes, and permanent vision damage. According to Dr. Richard Passwater, a world-renowned biochemist and nutrition expert, the reduction of glycation reactions and free radical production reduces the incidence of aging, heart disease, cancer, and arthritis.[3]

Fighting Back: Antioxidants Against AGES and Aging

Though the fairy tale of agelessness is alluring, we can't live forever. Nor can we look like we're twenty-nine years old forever either. With all that we know about human biochemistry and natural medicine, we can definitely slow down the process and stay younger longer, particularly in terms of our invaluable cardiovascular system. The solution is obvious: reduce the consumption of simple sugars and refined carbohydrates of all types that rapidly convert to glucose and enter the bloodstream. Consume antioxidant-rich foods and antioxidant supplements to prevent free radical damage.

Diabetics are much more susceptible to free radical damage than nondiabetics. Abnormally elevated glucose levels, typically found in diabetics, will oxidize and generate large quantities of free radicals. A study by A. Sharma and his colleagues demonstrated that vitamin E supplements taken in a daily dose of 400 IU (international units) decreased free radical damage, thus reducing the risk of diabetic complications.[4] Take antiglycation supplements (alpha-lipoic acid, chromium, bitter melon, and biotin) to control and normalize blood sugar levels. Exercise regularly. This will burn and clear glucose from the blood, summoning glucagon at the same time to bring glycogen and fats back into the blood so they can be burned for energy. Reduce stress.

Where's the Sweet Stuff?

Sugars are present everywhere in the diet, cleverly hiding in more foods than can be imagined. Identify sugars and refined carbohydrates by reading food labels for these familiar and not so familiar forms.

Simple Sugars

agave syrup	lactose
corn syrup	levulose
evaporated cane juice	maltose
fructose	molasses
high-fructose corn syrup	sucrose
honey	sugar
invert sugar	turbinado sugar

Refined Carbohydrates

breads (white flour)	muffins (white flour)
cakes	pancake mixes
cereals (white flour)	pastries
cookies	white flour
crackers (white flour)	white rice

Many natural remedies are available to reduce the symptoms of diabetes and the cardiovascular damage it causes.

Gymnema Sylvestre This Ayurvedic herb is called "gurmar," which means sugar destroyer. *Gymnema sylvestre*, an effective herb containing gymnemic acids, induces the pancreas to secrete insulin and lower blood sugar. Gurmarin, also found in *gymnema*, inhibits the sweet taste response. *Gymnema sylvestre* is a first-choice nutraceutical diabetic therapy.

Chromium This is a tried-and-true diabetic therapy favorite for promoting normal blood sugar levels. Glucose tolerance factor (GTF) chromium, niacin-bound chromium, chromium picolinate, and chelated chromium are good sources. Research studies show that niacin-bound chromium is more readily absorbed than other forms and is very effective for promoting normal levels of blood sugar, cholesterol, and triglycerides while increasing energy.

Alpha-Lipoic Acid Lipoic acid balances blood sugar by improving glucose utilization and slows down the production of glucose. It is also a powerful antioxidant that thwarts the dangerous free radical damage caused by excess insulin circulating through the blood and excessive fat metabolism.

Bitter Melon (*Momordica charantia*) The fresh juice of this unripe fruit contains well-documented antidiabetic properties. Bitter melon boosts pancreatic beta cell activity and may lower plasma glucose levels. Charantin, the primary active substance in bitter melon, is a powerful hypoglycemic composed of mixed plant steroids that studies show possess greater efficacy than prescription drugs. Bitter melon also contains polypeptide P, an insulin-like substance that lowers blood sugar levels in Type I diabetics. It does not interfere with prescription medications.

Apple Pectin This is a soluble fiber obtained from the famous "one a day keeps the doctor away" fruit. The soluble fiber slows the entry of glucose into the bloodstream, which prevents the quick entry and spiking of insulin common in diabetes and other blood sugar disorders. Apple pectin is available in capsules and powders, but stick with the capsules, as the powder does not dissolve well in plain water or juice.

Zinc This essential mineral is a critical component of insulin, involved in all aspects of its production and function.

Magnesium Magnesium is an essential macromineral for insulin production and utilization.

NAC (N-Acetyl Cysteine) This precursor to gluthathione, a potent antioxidant, prevents free radical damage caused by unbalanced, excessive fat metabolism.

Biotin A B-complex vitamin, biotin is probably the most underutilized and poorly studied dietary supplement for the management of diabetes. It plays a major role in the control of blood sugar, insulin resistance, and other blood sugar disorders. Biotin increases insulin sensitivity and enhances the activity of glucokinase, an enzyme critical to the efficient first step in the utilization of sugar by the liver. This was the conclusion that A. Reddi and colleagues presented in a 1988 paper in *Life Sciences*.[5] Biotin levels in diabetics are typically low. When beginning supplementation with biotin, it is advisable to speak to your doctor if you are diabetic, as it will likely lower your insulin requirements.

Vitamins B$_6$ and B$_{12}$ These essential vitamins reduce and prevent diabetic neuropathy. B$_6$ (pyridoxine) is essential for the cross-linking of collagen that is typically defective in diabetics due to their inability to absorb vitamin C.

Potassium Potassium improves insulin sensitivity and lowers blood pressure.

Vitamin E This improves insulin sensitivity.

Quercetin This bioflavonoid, found in red onions and grapefruit, increases the duration of effectiveness and activity level of vitamin C. It has a stabilizing effect on cell membranes and actively counters the destructive action in diabetic retinopathy. Quercetin also promotes the secretion of insulin and is a potent inhibitor of sorbitol accumulation, particularly in the eyes of diabetics. Reducing sorbitol prevents diabetic retinopathy and macular degeneration.

Essential Fatty Acids (EFAs) Omega-3s from flax oil and GLA from borage or evening primrose oil relax and soften arteries, reduce inflammation, and prevent systemic neuropathy.

Onions and Garlic These foods lower blood sugar.

Fenugreek (*Trigonella foenumgraecum*) Defatted seeds prepared from this Indian spice have a high fiber and gum content and are rich in 4-hydroxyisoleucine, which stimulates insulin production. Fenugreek's soluble fiber augments the body's ability to handle blood sugar, stimulates cells to burn glucose, and slows the passage of food and glucose absorption, thereby preventing dangerous after-meal insulin spiking.

Vitamin C Similar in structure to glucose, it is absorbed defectively by diabetics. This causes weak arteries because of the inability to produce sufficient collagen and poor immune function because of a lack of antioxidant activity. Vitamin C is not recommended often enough as a diabetic therapy and should be suggested as a "must take" part of a natural diabetic therapy protocol.

Glucomannan Derived from the root of the konjac plant, glucomannan is a poorly understood yet highly effective nonglycemic fiber that slows the entry of glucose into the bloodstream and curbs appetite.

Vanadium Forms like vanadyl sulfate and bis-glycinato-oxo-vanadium (BGOV) help to lower blood sugar.

Affair of the Heart: The Diabetes/CVD Connection

It cannot be stated strongly enough that the effects of diabetes on the cardiovascular system are insidious, slow, and devastating. Remember that diabetics absorb very little vitamin C. Consequently, not enough collagen is produced, causing the arteries to become thin, inelastic, fragile, and easily ruptured. Heart attacks are the leading cause of death in diabetics and diabetics have three times the risk of a fatal outcome as those who do not have diabetes.

This deficiency of vitamin C prevents the aggressive and effective quenching of free radicals. Not surprisingly, 33 percent of diabetics have high blood pressure and high cholesterol. There are other dangers, too. Excess sugar creates enormous volumes of urine that impart tremendous strain on the kidneys. Lack of glucose causes neuropathies that wreak havoc on the nervous system.

Sweet No-Nos

Avoid refined sugars, such as evaporated cane juice, honey, molasses, sucrose, corn syrup, high-fructose corn syrup, invert sugar, levulose, and turbinado sugar, and white flour foods, such as breads, muffins, pancake mixes, and cookies, as much as possible. Even though many of these items will be natural, all will create dangerous, potentially life-threatening fluctuations in blood sugar levels.

Take a Look at the Sweet Side

We've all got some sort of sweet tooth. It's a taste that is undeniably very pleasing, and for many it's addictive. We consume way too much sugary stuff. For cardiovascular health, it is imperative to dramatically lower the amount of sugar we consume. Try these excellent alternatives to sugar or artificial sweeteners for great-tasting nonglycemic sweetness. They are all natural, not chemically processed, and do not have the potential health dangers of artificial sweeteners.

Lo Han Kuo An extract of the Chinese herb Lo Han Kuo is available as HerbaSwee. According to its developer, Dr. Zhou of HerbaSway, HerbaSwee Lo Han Kuo is nonglycemic (glycemic index rating of less than 1), two hundred times as sweet as sugar, and has no calories. A great choice for diabetics!

Stevia (*Stevia rebaudiana*) This is a natural extract from the South American (sweetleaf) chrysanthemum native to Paraguay. This plant extract is noncaloric, nonglycemic (glycemic index rating of less than 1), and is available as a loose powder, powder packets, or liquid form ready to use in food.

Agave Syrup This delicious natural sweetener has a consistency that is slightly thinner than honey. It is naturally extracted from the agave cactus plant, native to the American Southwest, and retains its natural mineral content. Agave has a very low glycemic index of 11 and will not spike insulin levels unless you are diabetic; an excellent sweetener.

EFA Deficiency: Fat Facts and Fantasies

Essential fatty acids (EFAs) are critical for good health. Every cell in the body depends upon them to function properly. Cells in the heart muscle and cardiovascular tissues are especially needy. EFAs, part of every cell membrane, regulate nutrients and oxygen entering the cell and carbon dioxide along with other waste products exiting the cell. We are all confused about how much fat to eat and what types of fat to eat in our diets for heart health.

During the past decade there have been many low-fat and fat-free regimens offered to the public. Those diets, which advocated consuming lots of fat-free foods at a 5 to 10 percent fat level, focused solely on the amount, not the quality, of the fats consumed. The most important factor to consider when incorporating fat into the diet for optimum health is not the quantity of fat consumed but the type and quality of the fat consumed.

This critical fact, supported by the U.S. Surgeon General's report in 1988, stated that the type of fat we eat is one of the most significant factors affecting health and disease.[6] Low-fat diets at a level of 5 to 10 percent fat content, combined with "fat-free" foods can turn out to be unhealthy if the choice of fats is incorrect. However, a diet that incorporates a higher fat level of 15 to 25 percent can be extremely healthy if the types of fat consumed are the right ones.

> A heart-healthy regimen is rich in unrefined omega-3 and omega-6 fats.

The EFA Research Pioneers

In 1994, EFA expert Edward Siguel, M.D., of Boston University Medical Center, conducted research showing that patients with heart disease had biochemical evidence of EFA deficiency caused by insufficient levels of EFAs. Following that, he discovered that many Americans have a deficiency of essential fats. According to Dr. Siguel, consuming too much saturated fat compared to the amount of EFAs in the diet caused the deficiency, which he named EFAI (Essential Fatty Acid Insufficiency). Dr. Siguel then developed and patented a very sensitive technique with sophisticated instrumentation to measure levels of essential fats and deficiencies.[7]

How Much Fat Do We Need?

This is the great ongoing nutrition debate! According to some experts, at least .16 grams of essential fats per pound of body weight (24 grams for a 150-pound person) are required for health, in a ratio of anywhere from 4:1 to 10:1, omega-3 to omega-6 fats.

Dr. Siguel's suggested healthy ratio of omega-3 to omega-6 fats ranges from 1:4 to 1:10. He also indicates that a minimum amount of combined omega-3 and omega-6 EFAs be consumed daily. This is approximately ⅙ gram per pound of body weight or approximately 24 grams for a 150-pound person.

Based on extensive research, world-recognized fatty-acid expert Artemis Simopoulos, M.D., recommends consuming EFAs in a ratio varying from 1:1 to 1:4, omega-3 to omega-6. She explains that this is the best proportion with which our hunter-gatherer ancestors were genetically preprogrammed. Typical American diets have a ratio of omega-3 to omega-6 fats anywhere from 1:16 to 1:20. In other words, lots of omega-6 and virtually no omega-3! In fact, if you do not eat any fatty fish or dark green vegetables, you are not getting any omega-3s at all. And you're getting lots of omega-6, but not the kind you want. The omega-6 oils in the supermarket, such as generic vegetable, canola, or safflower oil, have been heavily processed with chemicals and exposed to air and light that oxidizes them. After processing, these oils no longer contain any healthy fatty acids, just rancid, oxidized fats, and contain none of the enzymes or vitamin activity that were originally present.

Understanding the Fat Facts

Fats are oily substances composed of carbon, hydrogen, and oxygen. They are the most concentrated source of food energy, containing twice as much energy (9 calories per gram) as carbohydrates and proteins (4 calories per gram each). Dietary fats are essential organic macronutrients that come from three primary sources:

- Plants, such as vegetables, legumes (beans), nuts, seeds and grains, avocados, and coconuts. Plant fats, typically rich in omega-3 and omega-6 EFAs (unsaturated fatty acids) or monosaturated fatty acids (the healthier types) and low in saturated fats/fatty acids (the unhealthy type), contain no cholesterol.

- Animal flesh, such as beef, pork, veal, chicken, turkey, and fish. Animal fats are typically just the opposite of the plant-source fats, being high in saturated fats (the unhealthy type) and low in unsaturated and monosaturated fats (the healthy type). They all contain cholesterol and break down to some extent into fatty acids that are precursors of inflammatory prostaglandins.

- Processed fats, such as vegetable oils, hydrogenated, and partially hydrogenated products, are not natural. They go through chemical processes to prevent spoiling and liquefying. This creates trans-fatty acids (TFAs) that are not as healthy as even the worst natural fats.

Fat-containing foods are complex mixtures of substances called fatty acids. Fatty acids are the components of fats and oils we derive from the foods we eat. Fat-containing foods do not contain merely one type of fatty acid in them, but rather a combination of the different types.

Fats are composed of three types of fatty acids. The type of fat is named according to the predominant fatty acid it contains. Butter, for example, is composed of 70 percent saturated fatty acids, so we call it a saturated fat. Olive oil is composed primarily of monounsaturated fatty acids, so we call it a monounsaturated fat. And flax oil, composed chiefly of polyunsaturated fatty acids, is called a polyunsaturated fat.

Fats in Your Food

Fat in food comes in a variety of forms, including the following.

The Benefits of Fats

- They provide the most concentrated source of dietary energy.
- They provide reserve energy when energy from glucose is not available.
- They are required for the production of hormones.
- They cushion and protect internal organs.
- They transport fat-soluble vitamins (vitamins A, D, E, and K) across the intestinal wall into the bloodstream.
- They lubricate joints and tissues and make the skin virtually waterproof.
- They are converted to essential fatty acids (EFAs), which are components of all cell membranes, regulating what goes in and out of every cell.
- The heart derives more than 50 percent of its energy from fats. Although natural fats are composed of three fatty acids, there are four basic types of fatty acids found in the diet because of unnatural TFAs (trans fatty acids) in margarines and other processed fat-containing foods.

PUFAs (Polyunsaturated Fatty Acids) Omega-3 and omega-6 fatty acids are the EFAs that you must get from your diet because they cannot be made in the body. They are critical for healthy metabolic and physiological development that begins from the time a fetus develops. Flax seeds, soybeans, walnuts, canola, and fish oils are excellent food sources of omega-3 and omega-6 fatty acids. The body produces derivative fatty acids from the two main precursor fatty acids in foods, omega-3 (alpha linolenic acid) and omega-6 (alpha linoleic acid).

There are three primary benefits of EFAs:

They regulate cell membrane function and fluidity.

They are precursors to localized hormonelike substances called eicosanoids (prostaglandins, leukotrienes, and thromboxanes).

They have enzymelike activities or become co-factors in enzymes.

Omega-3 Fatty Acids A team of researchers led by David S. Siscovick, M.D., attempted to assess whether dietary consumption of omega-3 fatty acids from fish was associated with a reduced risk of cardiac arrest. This valuable human study, using 334 people aged twenty-five to seventy-four, determined that consuming 5.5 grams of these fatty acids per month, equivalent to one fatty fish meal per week, reduced the risk of cardiac arrest by 50 percent![8]

The omega-3 fatty acid (alpha-linolenic acid—LNA) is predominant in flax seeds, its richest source. Via a sophisticated metabolic pathway, LNA is converted to two critical fatty acids, EPA (eicosapentaenoic acid) and DHA (docosahexanoic acid). DHA is a major component of cell membranes and critical for brain function. EPA keeps the blood thin and lowers triglycerides.

> ∞
>
> LNA (alpha-linolenic acid) >
> EPA (eicosapentaenoic acid)
> DHA (docosahexanoic acid)
> ▼
> eicosanoids: prostaglandins—
> thromboxanes—leukotrienes

Numerous studies have explored the cardioprotective effects of these essential fatty acids. Bruce Holub and Julie Conquer, at the Department of Human Biology and Nutrition Sciences, University of Guelph, Guelph, Ontario, conducted a DHA study in 1996. They set out to determine the effects of DHA blood values and the risk factors for heart disease in vegetarian populations by using an EPA–free algae source of DHA. The results of their study proved that DHA supplementation enhanced DHA blood levels, aided in the formation of EPA, and lowered both the total and LDL/HDL cholesterol ratios.[9]

Dietary DHA lowers triglycerides. In a 1997 study conducted by the Western Human Nutrition Research Center, San Francisco, California, the effects of DHA on fatty acids in tissue and plasma were studied. Consumption of DHA increased tissue levels of DHA and was able to lower triglycerides even without EPA present.

Omega-6 Fatty Acids Omega-6 fatty acids play numerous roles in cardiovascular health. Primarily, they are precursors to hormonelike substances called eicosanoids and prostaglandins that regulate hundreds of body functions. Omega-6 is the first step in the formation of GLA (gamma linolenic acid), a major inflammation fighter. By regulating membrane fluidity and function, Omega-6s control what goes in and out of cells and have a blood pressure–lowering effect.

The body uses these essential fatty acids in many different ways.

Eicosanoids and Heart Health Both omega-3 and omega-6 essential fatty acids are converted into substances called eicosanoids that affect cardiovascular function and health in many ways. There are three different types—prostaglandins, leukotrienes, and thromboxanes. Interestingly, they have some opposing effects.

PGE1 prostaglandins, derived from omega-3s, lower blood pressure with their vasodilating effects. They also control blood clotting by inhibiting the aggregation (clumping) of platelets. PGE2 prostaglandins, derived from omega-6

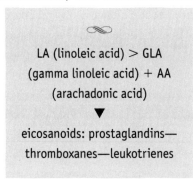

LA (linoleic acid) > GLA (gamma linoleic acid) + AA (arachadonic acid)

▼

eicosanoids: prostaglandins—thromboxanes—leukotrienes

EFAs, increase the permeability (leakiness) of vascular walls and cause inflammation. Overall, omega-6 fatty acids produce more inflammatory eicosanoids than omega-3 fatty acids. Thromboxanes, produced by omega-6 EFAs, are potent inducers of platelet aggregation and dangerous clotting that can cause heart attacks and strokes. Leukotrienes control your susceptibility to allergies and inflammation.

Monounsaturated Fats (MUFAs): Olive Oil and Heart Health

These are the nonessential fatty acids, called omega-7 (palmitoleic) and omega-9 (oleic acid). Omega-9 is found predominantly in olive oil. These days, there is great debate about whether olive oil can prevent heart disease. Your body can make MUFAs from saturated fats and it closely regulates their production. Levels of MUFAs can increase if we eat too many of them or if we eat too much saturated fat. When there is a deficiency of PUFAs, the body produces the next softest fat, MUFAs, to keep cell membranes soft.

Olive oil, rich in MUFAs, appears to lower the risk of cardiovascular disease by replacing hard saturated fats on the cell membrane in diets that are low in PUFAs. In some countries, the Mediterranean diet, plentiful in olive oil, appears to lower the risk of cardiovascular disease because it is consumed along with a healthy diet rich in PUFAs. Without sufficient omega-3 and omega-6 fats in our diets, olive oil, not the ideal fat for optimal cardiovascular health, would certainly be a better choice than the predominant, artery-clogging saturated fats and trans fats most of us consume.

According to Dr. Edward N. Siguel, M.D., in his book, *Essential Fatty Acids in Health and Disease*, by eating a dietarily benign monosaturated fat, such as olive oil, you may produce a softer, more flexible artery than by eating saturated fat. His premise is that the body uses monosaturated fat on the cell membrane to force out saturated fat derived from excessive saturated fat intake in the diet. He goes on to say that we appear to have the ability to make all the MUFAs we need, so they are unnecessary in our diets.[10,11] We suggest being conservative in the use of monosaturated fats from olive oil and stress the consumption of PUFAs from flax and other sources.

Saturated Fats (SFAs) At room temperature, saturated fats remain solid by comparison to PUFAs, such as flax and sunflower oil, or MUFAs, such as olive oil. Saturated fatty acids, in turn, are harder than PUFAs and MUFAs. When they take up space on the cell membrane, they incorporate their hardness and inflexibility to it. Cell membranes composed primarily of saturated fat will be hard and inflexible. This stiffness causes great resistance to blood flow, causing high blood pressure, and can accelerate the chance of damage or rupture. This stiffness also restricts nutrients and oxygen, particularly in heart cells, from entering freely and holds back metabolic wastes and toxins from exiting freely as well.

In all cases, the body seeks to achieve balance. Here it attempts to find the softest fatty acids it can for inclusion in the cell membranes. Diets high in saturated fats from meats, poultry, and dairy are also high in cholesterol and low in PUFAs. This forces the body to call out the softer fats. The natural one that can be made on demand is—cholesterol! Thus, cholesterol is a response to the harder fats present on the cell membrane.

If you consume hard, unhealthy saturated fats in your diet, your body will accumulate and incorporate hard, unhealthy saturated fats into your cell membranes.

Trans-Fatty Acids (TFAs): Margarine Myths and Toast with Real Butter!
Time was when everyone—including the doctor—said "margarine is good for you," making the claim that butter, because of all its saturated fat, was bad for your heart. Millions of us listened and ate margarine like it was going out of style. Oh, how wrong they were! Margarines are fake fats that have been manufactured in a food processing plant. Hydrogenated and partially hydrogenated margarines,

which have been the staple of the bread spread alternative to butter, are classic examples of scientifically engineered and altered fats that are rich in TFAs. The big problem here is that the body really does not recognize these chemically altered unnatural fats and has great difficulty removing them from the spots they take up on cell membranes and other sites in the body. Their inclusion on the cell membrane impedes the proper inflow of nutrients and oxygen, and the outflow of carbon dioxide and toxins.

All Fats Are Not Created Equal

Most of us think that fats are fats, right? Wrong! Don't allow yourself to be fooled by unknowing dieticians, doctors, educators, and government and industry organizations who tell you and want you to believe that all fats are created equal—meaning they contain lots of calories and nothing else. They haven't done their homework! And that means the wrong information for you.

Diets Rich in PUFAs Are Best

All the research conducted on fats concludes that diets rich in PUFAs provide the body with the greatest cardiovascular and general health benefits. Unadulterated PUFAs are the softest, most EFA– and nutrient-rich fats and are the natural choice for cell membranes. As it appears impractical for many of us and impossible for others to obtain all our PUFAs from dietary sources, we suggest taking EFA supplements.

Diets Rich in MUFAs Are Next Best

The next best thing to PUFAs in your food are MUFAs. The choice fat in this category is olive oil. Diets rich in olive oil as a main source of fat to complement rich amounts of PUFAs appear to be the healthiest diets in the world. The Mediterranean diet of the island of Crete in the 1960s is the classic example.

Diets Rich in SFAs Are Bad!

Saturated fats (SFAs) in the diet have been given a really bad rap and rightly so. They slow down your blood flow, increasing the chance of your blood clumping up. They are hard fats in food, and they remain hard fats in cell membranes. This hardness makes cell membranes stiff, inelastic, and rigid, more prone to injury than cell membranes filled with softer MUFAs and PUFAs. SFAs stimulate the production of cholesterol, which is a softer lipid for the cell membrane that replaces the hard fats.

Diets Rich in TFAs Are the Worst

TFAs are unnatural saturated fats that have been chemically altered by a process called hydrogenation. These fats are the worst offenders in your diet. You will see them referred to on food labels as hydrogenated and partially hydrogenated fats. Because of their unnatural chemical structure, the body does not recognize them with much ease and they clumsily fit into and disrupt cell membranes. This leaves the cell membranes hard, inflexible, and full of gaps, which affects nutrients and oxygen going in and carbon dioxide and wastes going out. TFAs also raise LDL cholesterol and lower HDL cholesterol. The FDA is now working to have food labels disclose the amounts of TFAs in foods. Read those labels. Don't eat margarines if they contain hydrogenated and partially hydrogenated fats!

Fats on You

All excess carbohydrates are converted to SFAs that are stored as body fat. Reducing stored SFAs—fat—depends on reducing dietary SFAs and the amount of food you eat. Dietary carbohydrates and sugars are converted into glucose. They become fats, too! In a nutshell, here's what happens to them. Glucose is burned for energy. When not required for energy it is converted to glycogen, a storage form of glucose stored in our muscle tissues. Excess glycogen in muscle is transferred into the liver and is stored there. When the liver is filled to capacity with glycogen, it overflows into the blood as triglycerides. Once the blood is filled with triglycerides, they exit the blood and are stored in adipocytes (fat cells that make up adipose tissue)—the fat on your body!

The body will also convert excess protein to body fat. All excess calories from all sources become SFAs and, consequently, adipose tissue. Excess food stimulates the production of SFAs. Excess saturated fats stimulate the production of a softer fatlike substance for the cell membrane. Without soft EFAs in the diet, the body produces more cholesterol, sending it to the cell membranes to keep them soft and flexible and thus excess circulating cholesterol.

How EFAs Prevent Heart Attacks

Statistics bear out that one out of two of us will die of some form of cardiovascular disease, unless we change the way we do things. Unfortunately, the odds are strong that you will have a heart attack or stroke whether you are male or female. While most women will be at much lower risk until after menopause because estrogen has a cardioprotective effect, epidemiological (population) data show that more women have heart attacks than men.

EFAs do a number of things to prevent heart attacks.

- They lower blood pressure.
- They do not convert into the dangerous, constricting eicosanoid thromboxane a2, but rather into thromboxane a3, which has only mild constricting power.

- Omega-3 fatty acids increase the production of nitric oxide, a potent vasodilator.[12]
- Omega-3 fatty acids have anti-inflammatory properties similar to aspirin but without irritation to the stomach lining.[13]
- One study reported that in men who ate fatty fish, 42 percent were less likely to die from a heart attack than those who did not eat fish at all.[14]
- EFAs, particularly omega-3 fatty acids, slow the formation of blood clots.[15]
- Omega-3s also make platelets less sticky, lowering the chance that they will clump together and block blood flow. Omega-3s decrease the production of fibrinogen, which becomes the fibrin in a clot that is held together by platelets.[16]
- EFAs have also been shown to prevent arrhythmias.[17]

A word of caution: Excess omega-3s can thin the blood and reduce its normal clotting activity. Excess omega-6s can increase dangerous blood clotting activity. American diets, overloaded with processed, useless omega-6s, are a major cause of blood clots.

Obesity: More Than a Battle of the Bulge

Being overweight causes body tissues to respond abnormally to insulin, forcing the pancreas to produce more than is normally necessary. Because insulin and, consequently, glucose are not taken up by receptors effectively, insulin resistance occurs. Abnormal elevations in blood pressure, decreased removal of cholesterol, and accelerated deposition of cholesterol result. Your heart must work harder to carry the extra weight. Those who are more than 30 percent overweight are most likely to have heart disease, even without other risk factors.

How our weight is distributed on our bodies is also a determining factor for risk. Fat around the abdomen, causing a beer belly or apple shape, and fat around the hips, causing a pear shape, are two basic types of fat accumulation. The apple shape is associated with a higher risk of stroke and CVD, hypertension, elevated triglycerides, low HDL cholesterol, and high blood sugar. The common factor causing these two types of obesity is elevated insulin and insulin resistance.

TEN

Lifestyle

Stress: The Battle Against Burnout

One of the major risk factors for cardiovascular disease, particularly CAD, is a person's type of personality profile. Much has been discussed over the years about the type-A personality. What is it? Are you one? A classic type-A personality is a person who is unusually aggressive, very pushy, highly competitive, and always trying to one-up and outdo the other person. This person is usually impatient, has a "gotta have it now" attitude, and has an extreme sense of time urgency, always in a great rush. Compared to non-type-A behavior, type-A people are twice as likely to have a cardiovascular accident.[1,2] Several studies confirm these findings and one study illustrated that the more aggressively a person behaved, the higher his or her cholesterol levels were.[3] Another excellent long-term study from 1975 to 1995 demonstrated that worry and stress dramatically increased the incidence of heart attacks.[4]

Stress Kills

Stress causes the adrenal glands to produce adrenaline and cortisol, the most potent hormones generated by the adrenal glands. It's the primitive "fight or flight" response. Chronic, prolonged stress causes the pancreas to generate excess adrenalin and cortisol. These hormones do not clear from the blood fast enough, as should normally happen in the body's ancient preprogrammed fight or flight response to conflict.

Ancient man usually fought a battle or fled, which cleared these hormones from the blood. Modern man employs no biological mechanism to eliminate them, and so emotional stress generates extra adrenaline and cortisol, which linger in the blood too long, eroding artery linings and initiating the repair/atherosclerotic process. Elevated levels of adrenaline and cortisol raise blood pressure and heart rate. These increases, particularly in blood pressure, heighten the risk of disrupting and possibly dislodging plaques on the arterial wall. This can initiate a blockage. The action of adrenaline and cortisol causes magnesium depletion. As magnesium is released from cells and excreted into urine, the risk of vasospasm and poor cardiac muscle contraction is increased.[5] Type-A personalities produce more adrenaline and cortisol; consequently, more magnesium is depleted.[6]

We will discuss ways to control stress in chapter 14.

Oral Health, Bacterial Infections, and Heart Disease

Many bacterial and viral organisms, particularly bacteria in dental plaques and dental infections, can affect the heart. A 1989 study by cardiologists in Finland established the positive relationship between poor dental health and the increased occurrence of heart attacks and stroke. And a sixteen-year study in the United States, conducted between 1971 and 1987, established a positive relationship between periodontitis, the advanced form of gum disease that affects the supporting structures of the tooth, and coronary artery disease. The study used a specific test, called a BANA test, to detect the presence of harmful anaerobic (existing without oxygen) bacteria in plaques. The conclusion was that a positive score on the test, confirming the presence of the bacterium, was twice as likely to be found in people with coronary heart disease.

When bacteria migrate from the mouth to the cardiovascular system, they settle in the heart muscle, causing inflammation that can become chronic. Long-term inflammation of heart muscle causes destruction of vital tissues needed for effective contraction and efficient pumping of blood. Fibers of the heart muscle weaken. Many cases of bacterial/viral invasion lead to cardiomyopathy (muscle disease). This enlarges and stretches the cavities of the heart, lessens efficiency, and leads to congestive heart failure, which decreases oxygen and nutrient supply to heart muscle and the rest of the body.

Dental infections can initiate an inflammatory response that releases dangerous substances, such as LPS (lipopolysaccharides) and HSP (heat shock proteins), that have a damaging effect on the intima of blood vessels. Dental infections raise white blood cell counts and initiate chronic inflammation of gums and the growth of unhealthy bacteria that can migrate to the cardiovascular system. Systemic oral enzyme therapy can destroy the main types of bacteria that are related to heart disease.

Cytomegalovirus and *Chlamydia pneumoniae*

Dr. Joseph Melnick of Baylor College of Medicine in Houston, Texas, has studied these bacterial renegades for more than seventeen years. Lesions from diseased arteries are found to contain *cytomegalovirus*, a common form of the persistent herpes virus. And *chlamydia pneumoniae* has been implicated in triggering the inflammation of tissues lining blood vessels that causes plaques.

This belief was supported in an August 2000 episode of NBC's *Dateline*, when correspondent Stone Phillips spoke to P. K. Shah, M.D., at Cedars-Sinai Hospital in Los Angeles, California. Dr. Shah believes that many cases of heart disease and heart attacks are triggered by the bacterium *chlamydia pneumoniae*, which accelerates the buildup of plaque and increases white blood cell activity. He noted that many people who have heart attacks did not have any of the other risk factors, including high cholesterol. *Porphyromonas gingivitis*, *bacteroides forsythus*, and *treponema denticola*, other common bacterial species responsible for causing gum disease, also damage artery linings.

Dr. Raoul Garcia of the Boston, Massachusetts, Veterans Affairs Outpatient Clinic examined eleven hundred men over twenty-five years of age. All healthy at the start, those who had the worst gums had twice the heart attack rate and three times the stroke rate of those with healthy gums. The bacteria mentioned above have been found in the carotid arteries of those participating in the study.

Wobenzyme N, the best-known and most studied oral enzyme nutritional supplement, destroys bacteria that cause heart disease by stimulating the immune system to increase the formation of tumor necrosis factor (TNF) and interleukins 1-b and 6, which attack bacteria and viruses. Wobenzyme N also increases the activity of bug-gobbling macrophages by 700 percent and NK (natural killer cells) by 1,300 percent. It also reduces inflammation and CRP levels after dental work.

At the Ukraine Scientific Institute of Cardiology, Kiev, Dr. I. K. Sledsewskaja noticed a significant drop in total cholesterol, LDLs, and triglycerides, and a reduction in atherogenesis with systemic oral enzyme therapy.[7] Therapy with Wobenzyme N corrects suppressed immune status after a heart attack and reduces blood lipids. Take care of your mouth!

Exercise and Overexertion

The health benefits of regular moderate exercise, and perhaps some strenuous exercise, cannot be overemphasized. But we all know that too much of a good thing is never really good in the long run. Ever notice those crazed weekend warriors, sweating and breathing like they're going to die?

Exercising beyond the physical capacity of the heart, which increases heart rate beyond the safe range, will result in severe exhaustion of the heart muscle and possible lowered efficiency in the future. This exhaustion can also cause the heart to enlarge, requiring more work for it to function. Overexercising also overloads respiratory function. When you begin struggling to breathe while exercising, it is an urgent warning signal that you are not getting enough oxygen to burn energy. This means, among other things, that your heart is also starved of oxygen—very risky! And your body is burning vital muscle tissue instead of glucose or fat for energy.

After too much exercise, the immune system is also weak. And let's not forget those nasty free radicals. Exercise always produces them. Prolonged exercise will produce a flood of free radicals that can be quite destructive if not offset with sufficient quantities of antioxidants in food and supplement form. Be cautious.

Alcohol, Smoking, and Drugs—Dumb, Dumber, and Dumbest

Three potentially deadly habits contribute greatly to cardiac problems.

Alcohol

Following smoking, excess consumption of alcohol is the second most preventable cause of death.

When consumed in excess or when consumed chronically as in alcoholism, alcohol is a powerful toxin to all body tissues and a nasty cardioirritant that irritates endothelial cells. When consumed in small to moderate quantities, your liver, assuming it is functioning optimally, detoxifies and renders alcohol harmless. When 2 or more ounces of ethanol (the pure form of alcohol) is consumed daily, high blood pressure results. Large quantities of alcohol can produce arrhythmias (irregular heartbeats) and cardiomyopathy that cause enlargement and flabbiness of the left and right ventricles. As the muscle deteriorates, pumping efficiency is reduced and heart failure can result.

Nearly one-third of all cardiomyopathy cases are attributed to excessive drinking. From a dietary and metabolic viewpoint, alcohol is not totally converted to energy and so becomes triglycerides circulating in the blood. Excess triglycerides that are not converted back to glucose are stored in the body as body fat.

Smoking: Stop Now and Prevent Premature Death

Numerous research studies clearly point to the fact that smoking is a cause of cardiovascular disease and the most common cause of preventable death. Arteriosclerosis and atherosclerosis are greatly accelerated by smoking. This occurs because smoking depletes vitamin C from the blood and tissues. Consequently, smokers have a higher risk of CVD (cardiovascular disease) and heart attack.

Carbon monoxide, the toxic, noxious exhaust gas from car engines with which we are all familiar, is also a major by-product of cigarette smoke, along with nicotine and approximately four thousand more toxic chemicals. Over time, increased levels of carbon monoxide destroy endothelial cells and damage blood vessel walls. This constantly initiates the Cardiovascular Metabolic Repair Response.

Smoking also lowers HDL cholesterol while raising LDL cholesterol and triglycerides. Smoking elevates normal levels of fibrinogen, needed for blood clotting. This increases the risk of forming dangerous clots. Smoking also increases levels of catecholamines (neurotransmitters), such as adrenaline and noradrenaline. These, along with nicotine, raise blood pressure and heart rate. This places more stress on the heart and constricts the arteries, decreasing blood flow.

There's good news though. Cardiovascular and general health risks decline rapidly after the smoker quits.[8] Almost immediately, constriction of peripheral blood vessels, induced by nicotine, stops. After approximately eight hours, carbon monoxide levels are down and blood oxygen levels have returned to normal. Furthermore, the risk of having a heart attack begins to decline within twenty-four hours.[9] And there's more—within one year of smoking cessation, your chances of developing heart disease drop by 50 percent and the risk of heart disease after five to ten years is essentially the same as if you had never smoked at all. This effect is the same for men and women.[10]

Illegal Drugs: Death by Dumbness

One of the simplest ways to experience severe chest pain, have a heart attack, or die suddenly is to use cocaine. Whether it is injected, smoked as crack, or just casually snorted, it only takes one use to possibly kill yourself or do irreparable damage to your heart. If you have any under- lying heart disease, diagnosed or not, your first high just might be your last. Cocaine leaves a nasty trail of destruction. It constricts blood ves- sels, accelerates heart rate, raises blood pressure, makes platelets more likely to clump, disrupts heart rhythm, and binds directly to heart mus- cle cells, impairing their normal function. Other illegal drugs, such as heroin, methamphetamine ("speed"), and mescaline can cause similar outcomes or death.

PART III

The Healthy Heart
Program

TO ACHIEVE OPTIMUM CARDIOVASCULAR AND WHOLE BODY
wellness, there are four primary areas you will need to consider:
diet, exercise, supplementation, and lifestyle modification.

1. **Diet:** This is the key to cardiovascular health. A balanced,
   lifelong eating program filled with heart-healthy foods that
   are rich in antioxidants, EFAs, vitamins, and minerals will
   provide most of what a healthy heart requires. Natural,
   unprocessed, well-balanced, varietal foods will also give you
   lots of energy to do the exercise you need to keep your heart
   strong. Many nutrients in food also promote healthy brain
   function, which will create a positive mental state essential to
   reducing stress and high blood pressure. So, food is much
   more than just energy to pump blood, breathe, move, and do

work. It has a major impact on everything else that occurs in the body. In addition to eating the proper foods and deriving the maximum benefit from their nutrients, it is most important to know that no matter how healthy a regimen you undertake, you will not get all the nutrients you need from food.

2. **Supplements:** For maximum cardiovascular health and protection, supplementation is a must! While there are many supplements that you can take, the most important ones should be taken every day.

3. **Exercise:** Regular exercise will strengthen your heart and make it pump more efficiently. It will also increase your metabolic rate and improve the utilization and efficiency of glucose. Exercise will increase the efficiency of respiration, enabling your lungs to process more air, meaning more oxygen for your heart. Finally, exercise produces chemicals called endorphins that have a calming effect, reduce stress, and keep blood pressure normal.

4. **Stress reduction:** Daily use of our stress reduction techniques, called the Serenity Prescription (see pages 236–239), will calm your body, lower your raging anxiety levels, and lower your blood pressure and heart rate. This will control factors that can trigger a dangerous cardiovascular event.

ELEVEN

Diet and the Healthy Heart

"Let food be thy medicine, and thy medicine be thy food."
—HIPPOCRATES

Diet Faddism

It could be the Atkins diet, the Carbohydrate Addict's diet, the Zone, or Protein Power. It could be the Pritikin diet, the Eat More Weigh Less diet, the McDougall Program, Stop the Insanity, FatBusters, or so on without end. Frankly, we could write a book about diet books. Despite the fact that each one presents itself as the unique, only true way to lose weight and be healthy, all have one thing in common: an extreme approach. And it's not a good thing. Extremism in your diet and nutrition planning is a recipe for poor health and emotional disaster. The promises are too big. The premises are too weak. The regimens are too restrictive. The long-term effects are not totally healthy.

And in many cases the results vary because of biochemical individuality or don't last because of noncompliance. Thin for life becomes fat again in no time at all!

The medically unsound, high-protein, ketogenic diet faddism programs and the fat-free extremes are partially right and partially wrong in their approach to weight loss. The wrong part is what will jeopardize your health. And it seems like there's a new diet fad every week. One that's guaranteed to make you lose weight and look and feel great. A few of these have emerged over the years and have captured the interest and pocketbooks of consumers.

But are they healthy? We don't think so, and here's why. In the last thirty years, hundreds of books have been written on the subject of so-called "healthy" diets. These diets range from complete fasts to single-food diets, from high-fat to no-fat diets, from high-protein to high-carbohydrate diets, and others, each trying to convince us that its way was the one guaranteed weight-loss and health-promoting program. One thing is quite clear: Diet extremism is very UN-healthy!

In any one given week or month, millions of people start a diet with the goal in mind to lose weight quickly and permanently. Let's examine the basic premise, biochemistry, benefits, and drawbacks of these different programs.

High-Protein Diets

Is too much protein dangerous? Most of the high-protein diets emphasize the excessive, disproportionate consumption of animal proteins, which contain unhealthy fats. Protein excesses from lots of beef, chicken, pork, veal, cheeses, and eggs shift the focus and function of two vital organs, the kidneys and the liver. The critical activities of these two organs are diverted from their required functions. Consequently, they increase in size over time from the constant overwork of processing excess proteins. As a result, they become much less efficient, and a highly toxic internal ecology results. Kidney stones (from excess urea generated by excess protein) and osteoporosis (due to calcium depletion from the bones that excess protein causes) are the result.

People with already compromised health status risk even greater danger. Certain proteins, like those from dairy, are in many cases highly allergenic. Dr. McCully points out in his book, *The Homocysteine Revolution*, that plant proteins contain significantly much less methionine than animal proteins. This strongly suggests that we can limit the body's potential to form excess harmful homocysteine from high levels of methionine by controlling the quantity of animal protein consumed in the diet. It also explains why populations that consume a plant-based diet are relatively protected against arteriosclerosis and atherosclerosis. This is in contrast to populations that consume a diet rich in meat and dairy products that afford minimal protection and high risk. Lower dietary levels of methionine generate lower levels of homocysteine, requiring less metabolic work and less folic acid, B_6, and B_{12} to convert homocysteine back to methionine. When we consume animal-based diets rich in beef, pork, poultry, and dairy, the need for folic acid, B_6, and B_{12} increases dramatically to accomplish this task.

How Much Protein Is Enough? Not as much as you think! The World Health Organization (WHO) and Dr. Linus Pauling, Nobel Prize–winning biochemist, suggest that .5 grams of protein per kilogram of body weight, equivalent to .36 grams per pound of body weight, is sufficient to provide enough building-block amino acids for growth and repair. For a 150-pound person, that represents approximately 54 grams, just about 2 ounces of protein per day. Infants, growing children, pregnant women, the elderly, those who are ill, and athletes typically require more protein.

Then There's the Fat Eating all you want of fat will make you fat. You will be consuming many more fat calories than necessary to maintain health. Your digestive system will be taxed more than normal. And you will certainly not be getting all the essential fats you need. Many animal proteins, such as beef and other meats, are typically treated with nitrites that combine with other substances called amines to form nitrosamines. These substances are carcinogenic compounds that can have devastating long-term effects.

Animal proteins are typically high in saturated fats which, if pre-dominant in the diet, become predominant in cell membranes, caus-ing stiffness and compromised integrity. Excess fats also cause the blood to clump, potentially clogging an artery in a healthy person, and certainly more likely to clog the arteries of a person with some level of undiagnosed cardiovascular disease. This will very likely cause a heart attack or stroke in someone who has visible signs of CVD (car-diovascular disease) or CAD (coronary artery disease). Unfortunately fad-diets only emphasize the quantity of fat, not the quality. They do not provide the heart-healthy omega-3 fats.

Without omega-3 fats, the body cannot make important fatty acid derivatives, such as EPA and DHA, and will not produce essential heart-healthy anti-inflammatory substances. These high-fat diets con-tain excess processed omega-6 fats. Consequently, the body will make too much of the unhealthy inflammatory substances, such as PGE2 prostaglandins and blood-clotting thromboxanes.

And Where's the Fiber? High-fat animal protein diets that are low in carbohydrates lack the fiber that is essential to proper, timely diges-tion. Fiber is also responsible for removing excess fats in the diges-tive tract that can be reabsorbed. One major shortcoming of high-fat diets is that they do not contain fiber, a disaster for your digestion. This slows down the digestive process, causing toxins to build up in the digestive tract.

No Plant Foods—No Antioxidants! This is the major drawback to a high-fat or high-protein diet. When carbohydrates from fruits, veg-etables, legumes, and grains are rarely consumed, the level of available antioxidants in the blood is very low. This means you are getting very little, if any, protection against free radical damage, especially against oxidation of LDL (low-density lipoprotein) cholesterol. In these diets, vitamin C levels are also very low, preventing the body from making sufficient collagen to build and maintain strong arteries.

High-Carbohydrate/Low-Fat Diets

For a while there was a fat-free craze. The message being broadcast stated that fat was unhealthy and basically unnecessary for your health. The logic of ultra–low-fat diets fed into the philosophy of the USDA food pyramid that suggested fats and oils had no nutritional value except for calories and that they should be used sparingly. Several of the low-fat diets advocated fat levels of 5 to 10 percent, claiming more was very dangerous, especially for people with heart disease.

Since these diets did not advocate high protein, the emphasis was on carbohydrates. But some of the diets were not clear about the type of carbohydrates that should be eaten, suggesting we eat all the pasta, rice, bread, and cereals we want. The error of this thinking is that these diets did not clearly differentiate between complex and refined carbohydrates.

Eating all you want of refined carbohydrates will raise your triglyceride levels. You will also consume far more calories than necessary to maintain a healthy weight. Your digestive system will be taxed more than normal. Because these carbohydrates have been stripped of their enzymes and minerals in the process of preparing them, they are nutrient-deficient, empty foods. They trigger the pancreas to produce more digestive enzymes than it should. These refined carbohydrates are void of fiber, which is a disaster for digestion.

The worst aspect of a diet high in refined carbohydrate foods is that these foods yield unhealthy amounts of simple sugars. When dietary fats or proteins are replaced with simple carbohydrates, more fast-entry, insulin-spiking glucose enters the blood. Excess insulin creates hypoglycemic cycles, which stimulate appetite and negative mood changes. Higher levels of glucose in the blood means more glycogen formation in the muscles and the liver. The excess glycogen in the liver, in turn, spills over into the blood as triglycerides. If not converted back to glycogen and glucose, they become adipose tissue— body fat. The excess glucose circulating in the blood, as discussed earlier, will bind to proteins in the artery walls. This process, called glycation, will damage the collagen and cause arterial injury. This initiates the cardiovascular metabolic repair response of inflammation, immune response, deposition of lipoprotein(a), cholesterol and more. A vicious cycle begins. But you can break it.

Eat Smart for a Healthy Heart

There's no big mystery about how to develop a healthy eating style that is tops for your heart and unsurpassed for the rest of your body. Diet should not be a chore or viewed as a restrictive event. Rather, it should be an enjoyable, varietal, tasty experience that naturally develops into a lifestyle over time.

This is the wisest way to eat because we are unaware of which nutrients we need at any given time unless we can take specific, expensive tests. The grim reaper waiting to take your heart in small pieces is disguised in unhealthy food and the poor, impulsive, and often lazy choices we make when deciding what to eat.

The healthiest diets for the long term contain a wide variety of nutrient-dense foods.

Healthy Diets Around the World

In many other cultures, people live longer, healthier lives than we do here. Why? In each diet, certain foods consumed on a regular basis are extremely healthy. We compared some of these healthier diets and found some common food denominators that optimize wellness.

The Mediterranean Diet This is the Greek diet of the island of Crete as it was in the 1960s. People there consumed lots of fresh, local fruits, vegetables, grains, and nuts that never sat in warehouses and cold storage, losing vitamin content by the minute. The foods were free of sprays and chemicals. Fresh breads were made from locally grown and freshly milled whole grains. Locally caught fish was eaten fresh the same day. Freshly made cheeses were produced without additives. Occasional small quantities of butchered meats were eaten, from free-range animals raised locally without chemical maintenance. Garlic was used every day. Low–alcohol content red wine was consumed frequently. Almost no refined sugar or carbohydrates were consumed. No processed oils were used, just fresh-pressed olive oil along with other nut and seed oils. Trans fats did not exist.

The Japanese Diet The traditional Japanese diet is a mix of good and bad foods. On the good side, there is a major emphasis on fresh vegetables and fruit. Soy is a central part of the diet and represents a significant proportion of its protein. The diet is low in saturated fat, with animal protein coming primarily from fish. Garlic and ginger are consumed every day. Green tea, high in the most potent antioxidants known to prevent free radical damage and oxidation of fats, is consumed in large volumes. The diet is low in refined sugars. However, the Japanese diet is loaded with miso, soy sauce, and other salty foods. White rice, the primary carbohydrate, has no fiber and rapidly raises blood sugar. Despite that, the Japanese have about half the rate of heart disease than in the United States.

The French Diet The French paradox—better health while consuming more fatty foods and smoking lots of cigarettes—is something not everyone understands. Here's one clue: The diet is very low in unhealthy refined sugars and carbohydrates that promote glycation and insulin resistance. Unprocessed oils, such as olive oil, are regularly used. TFA–rich margarines or processed oils are not consumed.

Locally produced, freshly made butter and cheeses without additives are regular choices. Whole grain breads, not refined white breads, are eaten daily. Red wine, rich in polyphenol antioxidants, is commonplace at the table. And we know now that it is not the alcohol, but the polyphenols in the wine that protect the heart.

The Paleolithic Diet This is the diet that was consumed by ancient man. At that time, humans were hunter-gatherers, roaming about for food to sustain their lives and shelter to protect them from the elements. They hunted birds, animals, and when near water, fished whenever possible. Sources of these foods were very irregular. When available, they were fresh, untainted with chemicals and processing. Ancient humans also foraged; they gathered fruits, berries, nuts, vegetables, honey, leaves, and tree bark for food, depending largely on local supplies. These were fresh foods, rich in vitamins, minerals, enzymes, essential fatty acids, and phytonutrients. Ancient man did not cultivate grains until about 8,000 B.C.

SAD: The Standard American Diet Status quo for most Americans is the Standard American Diet and it's been that way for decades. The Standard American Diet is in fact very sad! It is loaded with foods that have been bleached, deodorized, overprocessed, and refined. These foods are rarely fresh; storage and processing depletes and removes vital nutrients, enzymes, fiber, tastes, and textures. They are treated with a vast array of chemical additives, colorings, waxes, preservatives, and conditioners. They also contain drug residues, antibiotics, hormones, plus other toxins, and are packaged in containers that release harmful substances into your body and the environment, which damages your health and the ecology. These foods barely resemble their original forms.

Eating for a healthy heart means eating natural fresh foods that are "alive." These foods are brimming with vitamins, minerals, amino acids, essential fatty acids, fiber, food-digesting enzymes, phytonutrients, probiotics, and hundreds, perhaps thousands, of other health-promoting substances. These foods are freshly picked and are eaten raw or minimally cooked. They are free of toxic chemical additives, preservatives, waxes, colorings, and conditioners. They do not contain poisonous drug residues, antibiotics, hormones, or added toxins. Prepared natural foods are packaged in containers that do not release harmful substances and are ecologically safe. These foods are in their original forms.

How Each Diet Affects Your Health

The Standard American Diet is very destructive to the body and mind. It severely stresses all the body systems and organs by constantly making them work much harder than normal. The body must metabolize incoming substances that are not orthomolecular (natural) or recognizable to it. A chronically overworked body wears down more easily over time, needs constant repair, lacks the necessary resistance to disease, and must repair itself more often. As a result, it wears out much sooner, causing early-onset chronic illness, disease, and death.

In contrast, eating for a healthy heart builds optimal health, wellness, and resistance to disease by providing only food substances that are orthomolecular (natural) and recognizable to the body. It actively and aggressively supports body functions, eliminating the constant and severe metabolic stress caused by the "food garbage" that predominates in the Standard American Diet. Nutrients in the healthy-heart diet plan are more bioavailable to the cells and organs. Body systems have more energy to work at growth, repair, and immunity to disease at consistently more effective levels.

This diet is the healthiest for your cardiovascular and whole body health. It is a plant-based diet that is rich in natural foods from the following food groups:

- fruits
- vegetables
- starchy/root vegetables

- legumes (beans, especially soy)
- whole grains
- nuts and seeds
- unprocessed, healthy oils
- Omega-3–rich fish
- meat, poultry, eggs, and dairy (occasional or optional)
- pure water and clear liquids

These foods are low in artery-clogging saturated fats, yet naturally rich in heart-healthy omega-3 and omega-6 fats. They are also rich in antioxidants, vitamins, minerals, a broad range of phytonutrients like vitamin C, vitamin E, carotenoids and bioflavonoids, digestive enzymes (amylases, lipases, proteases, cellulase), and both soluble and insoluble fiber. These foods also contain a natural abundance of blood pressure–lowering potassium and are low in pressure-elevating sodium.

Just Say "No" to Extreme Cuisine

We strongly urge you to avoid the medically unsound ketogenic high-protein diet faddism of many diet programs offered today. Ketogenic diets (producing unhealthy substances called ketones, which result from excess protein consumption) are low in the artery-building antioxidant vitamin C. They are high in cholesterol. Ketogenic diets generate large amounts of uric acid from the metabolism of protein. They cause excess calcium excretion and frequently cause fatigue and hypotension.

On the opposite end of the diet spectrum, ultra–fat-free, highly refined carbohydrate diet extremes filled with pasta, rice, and breads should be avoided as well. These cause large spikes in blood sugar and insulin levels. They provide high levels of glucose that can bind to proteins in the artery wall, causing glycation and AGES. As a result, triglyceride levels jump up dramatically. And if you are consuming too many calories, a very likely scenario on these diets, you will gain weight. Promise yourself to ignore the false potential of quick-fix, fast–weight-loss diets. We know they are sure to put your body through nutritional and emotional hell. You will only gain back the weight when you tire of these diets. Then you will suffer the consequences of the diet's detrimental effects and find yourself even more unhappy and frustrated than before. The best lifelong diet is one in which there are healthful variations.

Eating for Heart and Whole Body Health

When beginning your diet for a healthy heart, set your sights on four goals that will maximize your cardiovascular health.

1. Keep blood sugar levels normal by reducing and eliminating refined carbohydrates and simple sugars.
2. Avoid extra calories. Maintain a healthy and trim weight by reducing your consumption of food, especially refined carbohydrates and simple sugars.
3. Get lots of nutrients rich in natural blood thinners, antioxidants, blood pressure–lowering bionutrients and natural chelating agents in your food by eating a wide variety of plant foods.
4. Keep blood pressure levels normal by achieving a much higher than typical potassium to sodium ratio.

Avoid Extra Calories: Maintain a Healthy and Trim Weight

Don't listen to anyone that tells you that you can eat all you want. It's a scientific fact that excess calories derived from food of any type are stored as fat. Extra calories in any form, whether they come from fats, proteins, or carbohydrates, will be converted into body fat.

One scientist, Dr. Roy Walford, has been studying the effects of what he calls undernutrition for years. That means eating less, much less than you think. Don't worry, you won't starve! His overall results: Animals and people live longer on less food. Much less digestive and enzymatic activity is directed towards digesting food and much more enzymatic activity is directed toward repair and growth.

Get Lots of Nutrients

The more the merrier! The most varied diet provides the most nutrients. Plant-based nutrition is rich in phytonutrients, vitamins, minerals, EFAs, live enzymes, fiber, and high-quality protein. Animal foods don't contain much in the way of vitamins, minerals, or EFAs. Nor is there any fiber in animal foods, making digestion much slower. The foods must be cooked to be eaten, so there are no live enzymes. The pancreas must make large amounts of digestive enzymes to digest them. Worst of all, animal foods do not have *any* phytonutrients. Absolutely none!

Natural Blood Thinners

Garlic, onions, leeks, and others in the allium family have proven blood-thinning properties. Use them liberally in fresh salads and cooked foods. Roast garlic for a delicious addition to soups, salad dressings, or as a spread.

Flax oil and ground flax seeds, the richest source of omega-3 fats, from a high-quality source, have a great, lightly nutty taste. They are terrific as your oil for salad dressing or on whole grain bread instead of margarine or butter, brushed over corn on the cob, or in mashed potatoes. Crushed flax seeds are excellent in whole grain bread mixes, mashed potatoes, brown rice, or sprinkled over salads. Because flax seeds and flax oil are heat and light sensitive, they should never be used as cooking oils. Flax seeds and oil should be refrigerated, and once the seeds are ground, keeping them in the freezer is best. Quality flax contains vitamin E and beta-carotene too.

Fish, particularly fatty fish such as salmon, mackerel, herring, and sardines, are also very rich in omega-3 fatty acids. Consume them regularly, at least one to three times weekly for maximum blood-thinning effects. Bake, broil, poach, or steam with your favorite sauces and veggies.

Foods That Lower Your Blood Pressure

To achieve a much higher than typical potassium to sodium ratio, consume a diet rich in plant foods, and low in animal foods and salt-laden processed foods. Instead of oversalting your food, season it with spices. To further lower your blood pressure, increase the potassium to sodium ratio in your diet by increasing the quantity and percentage of plant foods you eat.

In our previous discussions, we told you that high blood pressure can be lowered by changing the ratio of potassium to sodium in the blood. To accomplish this, simply change the ratio of potassium-rich foods to sodium-rich foods in your meals. Typical diets have a ratio of as much as 20 to 1—sodium to potassium—very salty! This is a definite reason for high blood pressure.

The Standard American Diet, the one you just might be on now, is filled with processed foods—canned soups; chips; pretzels; meats treated with sodium nitrite; condiments, such as ketchup, pickles, relishes, salad dressings; and canned vegetables. A diet that is healthy for your heart typically has a ratio of 4 to 1 to 20 to 1, potassium to sodium. That means lower blood pressure! This happens because plant foods are a major part of the diet and are naturally very high in potassium, while containing almost no sodium.

High-potassium foods to eat regularly include potatoes, bananas, orange juice, lima beans, raisins, spinach, apricots, and cantaloupe.

Eat Lots of Antioxidant-Rich Foods

Don't forget: Antioxidants are the body's "antirusting" substances— your biopolice working 24/7. They are free radical scavengers that prevent cell membrane damage. Antioxidants prevent the oxidation of fats, oxygenate the cells, and protect against the negative effects of foreign substances in chemicals in food, air, and water. They destroy carcinogens and stimulate immune system function.

Plant Foods Are Where the Antioxidant Action Is! The list of antioxidants for health and optimum wellness could fill volumes. Here are some suggestions:

- **Citrus fruits:** Oranges, grapes, lemons, limes, and kiwi provide lots of vitamin C and citrus bioflavonoids.
- **Melons:** Cantaloupe, papaya, guava, and watermelon provide lots of beta-carotene and lycopene.
- **Green foods:** Spirulina, chlorella, wheat grass, barley grass, kamut grass, wakame, and kombu are rich in chlorophyll.
- **Berries:** Blueberries, cranberries, boysenberries, blackberries, raspberries, and pomegranates are loaded with anthocyanidins, proanthocyanidins, resveratrol, and ellagic acid.
- **Grapes:** Red grapes, particularly Concord grapes, are rich in resveratrol, anthocyanidins, proanthocyanidins, polyphenols, and ellagic acid.
- **Vegetables:** Broccoli and cauliflower contain high amounts of indole-3-carbinol and sulforaphane. Peppers are rich in vitamin C. Garlic, onions, scallions, shallots, and leeks are filled with sulfur-rich antioxidants (s-allyl-cysteine, s-allyl-mercaptocysteine, and quercitin).
- **Root vegetables:** Potatoes, sweet potatoes, and yams are loaded with vitamin C, beta-carotene and other carotenes, magnesium, and other minerals.
- **Nuts and seeds:** Flax and walnuts are excellent sources of omega-3 and omega-6 fatty acids and isoflavones. All varieties are rich in vitamin E, tocopherols, and tocotrienols. Flax is especially rich in beta-carotene and vitamin E.
- **Whole grains:** The ancient grains—amaranth, quinoa, spelt, teff, kamut, and millet are supernutritious. All types of whole

grains are high in vitamin E, selenium, other minerals, and cholesterol-lowering phytosterols.

- **Legumes:** All varieties of beans are rich in vitamin E, selenium, isoflavones, and EFAs.
- **Green tea:** This is rich in polyphenols, especially EGCG (epigallocatechin gallate), which is reported to be two hundred times more potent than vitamin E and perhaps more potent than any other antioxidant.

Twelve Super Antioxidant Supplements

The following twelve antioxidant supplements will keep your cardio-vascular system young and healthy.

1. Alpha-lipoic acid is a unique water- and fat-soluble antioxidant capable of quenching many more free radicals than other water- or fat-soluble antioxidants. It regenerates vitamins C and E, while scavenging and destroying hypochlorous, peroxy, and hydroxy radicals.
2. Lycopene is the red carotenoid found in tomatoes, red grapefruit, apricots, and watermelon. This incredibly aggressive antioxidant has been the subject of much recent research positively validating its free radical–quenching and cancer-preventive abilities.
3. Indole-3-carbinol and sulforaphane stimulate the production of carcinogen-killing enzymes. They are plentiful in brussels sprouts, kale, collard greens, broccoli, mustard greens, cabbage, and cauliflower.
4. Alpha tocopherol is commonly known as vitamin E, one of eight forms found in the vitamin E complex. Four are tocopherols, possessing antioxidant activity that has been validated in thousands of studies. Four are tocotrienols, cousins to vitamin E, which support the activity of alpha tocopherol. Olives, nuts, and seeds are rich sources.

5. Vitamin C, found in citrus fruits, tomatoes, peppers, broccoli, and hot red peppers is the primary water-soluble antioxidant in the body. Thousands of studies clearly support vitamin C's ability to protect against free radical damage. Because we cannot produce vitamin C internally, we must obtain it from food and supplemental sources.

6. Beta-carotene is one of six hundred carotenes noted for their effectiveness at quenching singlet oxygen and other free radicals.

7. Vitamin A, the "anti-infective," maintains skin, respiratory tract surfaces, mucous membranes, and secretions, thereby reducing free radical activity generated by infection. Vitamin A converts from beta-carotene in the liver, stimulating production of white blood cells.

8. Lutein, discovered in marigolds, is the eye antioxidant that prevents macular degeneration.

9. Beta 1,3 glucans is a yeast-derived carbohydrate from the cell wall of baker's yeast, stripped of protein to prevent yeast allergies and stripped of fat to ease absorption. Another type of beta 1,3 glucans is derived from an organically grown mushroom known as *Agaricus blazei murill*, a rare Brazilian fungus. Both sources of beta-glucans provide powerful immune system support by activating and stimulating the immune system to produce large quantities of macrophages and natural killer cells. These specialized cells in the immune system attack and engulf dangerous invading pathogens.

10. NAC (n-acetyl cysteine) is an amino acid derivative that is a precursor to gluthathione, the essential and most effective antioxidant in the liver.

11. SOD (superoxide dismutase) is an antioxidant enzyme that prevents damage from the superoxide radical.

12. Red/purple grapeskin contains compounds called *polyphenols* that have extremely high antioxidant values and especially

high free radical–quenching abilities. The cardiovascular protection that red/purple grape polyphenols confers is virtually unmatched. One study reportedly showed red/purple grape juice more effective than 40 fruits and vegetables tested.

Put Old Age in the Back of Your Mind

We all want to live forever, but know we can't. Get your fountain of youth arsenal together today. Go straight to your favorite green grocer or supermarket for those "turn back the clock" antioxidant foods. Eat five to ten servings of fruits and vegetables each day. Have a refreshing green drink. Munch those prunes. And drink your grape juice. A glass a day keeps old age away!

Super Soy for Peak Heart Health

As recently as ten years ago, American farmers grew the lowly soybean almost exclusively as feed for pigs, cows, and chickens. Then perhaps, a few health nuts, vegetarians, and those with food allergies ate some tofu and drank some soymilk as part of their diets. Not so anymore. Soy-based foods are leaping forward as the hottest food category of the new millennium.

Nutritional Allure and Culinary Magic Soy is a nutritional powerhouse dietary supplement and versatile culinary ingredient that is recipe friendly and tasty to the palate. Soy has found its way into dozens of different food categories and forms—supplements, snacks, shakes, and meat substitutes—that were previously unimaginable.

The rising popularity of soy foods is driven by consumer demand that is increasingly sophisticated. All types of soy foods are a perfect fit for the health conscious, vegetarians, vegans, people with dairy allergies, infants and toddlers, those who don't eat meat because of religious beliefs, and the newest and fastest-growing category—the curious. And curious they are. Seventy-one percent of people are already aware that soy is healthy, and 50 percent know why. Tasty, pre-cooked, versatile meat alternatives are perfect recipe substitutes for the 60 percent of the population that wants to lower consumption of meat. Yet only 20 percent of people actually do it because they don't want to miss the satisfaction of meat in their diet.

Soy owes much of its skyrocketing consumption to the fact that it is provably health promoting. In October 1999, a health claim made for soy was accepted and approved by the FDA. This claim specifically states that 25 grams of soy protein a day, as part of a diet low in saturated fat and cholesterol, may reduce the risk of heart disease.

Welcome to Soy World! Soy is one of few foods to receive FDA approval to make a health benefit claim. Here's a list of soy foods so comprehensive, it will be impossible for you not to eat some practically every day and love it, too. Some of our favorites are below:

> **Edamame:** It's the latest soy food rage! These large fresh green soybean pods cooked in salted water are crunchy, sweet, and delicious as side dishes or between-meal snacks.
>
> **Meat alternatives:** Textured soy protein (TSP) is chunks or granules of defatted soy. This ultra–low-fat protein looks and cooks like its ground meat competitor. TSP absorbs all types of seasonings and is fantastic for making chilies, "meat" sauces, and sloppy Joes. Soyburgers look and taste just like the real thing when you slide them on the bun! Soydogs and flavored sausage are super on a bun, too. Do you like cold cuts? Pick up some salami, turkey, and ham style, as well as other deli meat substitutes made from the bean. How about bacon? Try some scrumptious soy with the sizzle and taste of the real thing for your next BLT or scrambled eggs breakfast, without the fat or cholesterol.

Miso: The traditional Japanese fermented soybean paste with an intense salty flavor comes in light to dark varieties for seasoning a variety of foods such as soups and dressings.

Natto: These fermented, cooked whole soybeans have a nice, cheesy texture and make great toppings for rice and vegetables.

Nondairy soy frozen desserts: Ice cream, watch out! Frozen soy desserts are a delicious alternative.

Soy cheese: These first-rate stand-ins for dairy cheeses are available in delicious traditional or flavored meltable slices.

Soy flour: Soy flour is made from roasted soybeans milled into a fine powder that can be introduced as a baking alternative with an isoflavone and protein boost. Replace some of your regular, unhealthy white flour (about one-third to one-half the volume) with heart-healthy soy flour.

Soy grits: Toasted and coarsely cracked soybeans become high-protein grits to cook along with rice and grains or to prepare alone for a healthy, belly-warming breakfast cereal.

Soy sauce: Also known as tamari, shoyu, and teriyaki, these dark brown liquid sauces in regular or aged gourmet varieties are zesty seasonings for all types of foods.

Soy yogurt: This creamy dairy alternative is offered in tangy fruit flavors that have the look, mouth feel, and taste of the real stuff. You might not taste the difference.

Soymilk beverages: This soy staple, prepared from soaked, ground, and strained soybeans, is high in protein, B vitamins, and isoflavones. It's got calcium, too! Regular and lite varieties are ideal for making delicious creamed soups, and soymilk is a tasty substitute for milk in breakfast cereals or pancake mixes. Flavored soy milks (carob, chocolate, vanilla) make scrumptious shakes and smoothies.

Soy nutrition bars/shake powders: Nutrition bars are flying off the shelves faster than ever. Shoppers are grabbing soy-based bars when there's no time to make their favorite shake. Meal replacement shake powders without the usual junk in them are available to satisfy the palate in great-tasting gourmet flavors when the urge strikes.

Soynuts and butters: Roasted whole soybeans in salted, unsalted, and seasoned versions are the crunchy snack that easily rivals those tired old roasted peanuts. They are also ground into creamy or chunky-style spreads—move over peanut butter!

Soybean oils and salad dressings: The most widely consumed oil in the United States, soybean oil is used for cooking and as a base for salad dressings. Purchase only unrefined, expeller-pressed soybean oil and products.

Tempeh: A traditional Indonesian food, this chunky, tender, fermented soybean cake with a smoky, nutty flavor makes a great entrée food when marinated and grilled, or added into your favorite casseroles or chilies.

Tofu: This soymilk standard (also called soybean curd) is a soft cheeselike food curdled from fresh hot soymilk. Tofu is practically tasteless and easily absorbs the flavors of the ingredients with which it is cooked. Produced in several forms, each is suited for various cooking techniques and recipes.

Yuba: This more obscure soy food is the thin surface layer of cooling hot soymilk, sold in sheets, either fresh, half-dried, or dried. Yuba makes great wraps for tacos and tamales, and a replacement for sheet pasta.

Soy sprouts: These are a crunchy addition to salads, sandwich toppings, soups, and stir-frys.

Other great soy foods: Soy mayonnaise is a flavorful mayo substitute for spreads, dips, and salads without the cholesterol. Or how about a soy pizza to satisfy that urge?

Got chips? Put some crunchy soy snack chips on the coffee table to munch with those dips.

What About GMOs?

Soy is the new health food rage, but can we count on it to be GMO (genetically modified organism) free? Not yet, say the experts. Although a growing number of soy supplements and food products are already GMO free, we can't clearly know without testing whether they're tainted or not. How to know for sure? Manufacturers are beginning to buy their beans from certified GMO-free crops and test them via certification labs. Then they can clearly and confidently label their products as third-party certified GMO free.

As for organic soybeans, it is also incorrect to assume that they are definitely GMO free simply because they are organic. While it's less likely that organic soy products contain GMOs because organic producers are considerably more concerned about unnatural substances in or on the beans and their growing environment, this is still no guarantee. Nature's simple process of cross-pollination can transfer GMOs from one crop to another quite easily. Make sure your foods are labeled GMO free.

Chocolate: Sweet Nutrition for a Healthy Heart

Would you believe that chocolate is healthy for your heart? This heavenly treat was first discovered by Europeans on the fourth voyage of Columbus in 1502. Those phytonutrients have done it again. This time it's the antioxidants found in the cocoa bean that are causing this excitement.

Numerous studies show that the levels of polyphenols (epicatechin and catechin) found in cocoa powder extract, the same ones found in green teas and wine, were extremely high. According to Andrew

Waterhouse of the Department of Viticulture and Enology at the University of California, Davis, California, a cup of hot chocolate using two tablespoons of cocoa had 146 mg of polyphenols, compared to a 1.5-ounce bar of milk chocolate at 205 mg polyphenols. This can be compared to a 5-ounce glass of red wine, which contains 210 mg of antioxidant phenols. And cocoa powder turned out to be a potent cardioprotective antioxidant against LDL oxidation, which forms deadly oxidized LDL cholesterol. Apparently, cocoa is a more potent antioxidant than red wine. Plus, cocoa is rich in heart-healthy magnesium too.[1]

TWELVE

Supplements for Cardiac Health

WE'VE TALKED ABOUT THE MANY MISCONCEPTIONS THAT surround the onset and development of cardiovascular and coronary artery disease. And we've laid out the real causes. We've explained how the body responds to arterial injury, how it controls fats and cardioirritants in the blood, and how it maintains efficient blood pumping and flow. By now we hope you have learned precisely what a heart-healthy diet looks like in practical terms.

But as we mentioned earlier, no matter how perfect your diet and no matter how well you eat, you will definitely not get all the nutrients you need from food because most American diets are self-limited to about twenty basic foods with little variation beyond that. The levels of nutrients critical to maintaining a healthy heart and whole body are absolutely not present in food, organic or not.

The bottom line is this: Sensible supplementation is essential for healthy cardiovascular function and healthy function of the heart, circulatory system, and blood. Our next step is to tell you about the dietary supplements you must take for maximum cardiovascular health. These include the newest, cutting-edge dietary supplements and their incredible effects on cardiovascular and whole body health, and the tried and true ones, too.

Quick Guide to Cardiac Health

The following is a quick guide of supplements strategies to reduce risk factors and promote maximum cardiovascular health.

1. **To improve cardiac efficiency and energy:** Hawthorn, co-enzyme Q10, l-carnitine, d-ribose, chlorophyll, coenzyme A (as the pantethine form of B_5).
2. **For healthy cell membranes and cell membrane integrity:** omega-3 and omega-6 essential fatty acids, flax, EPA.
3. **To lower homocysteine:** Vitamin B_6, vitamin B_{12}, folic acid, TMG (trimethylglycine), and choline.
4. **To lower lipoprotein(a):** Niacin (as nicotinic acid), l-lysine, l-proline.
5. **To lower blood lipids:** EFAs, niacin (as inositol hexaniacinate), artichoke extract, guggulipid, vitamin C, red yeast rice, phytosterols, soy, garlic.
6. **To normalize blood sugar:** Guggulipid, artichoke, niacin as inositol hexaniacinate, phytosterols, EFAs, chromium, bitter melon, biotin, zinc, magnesium, vanadium, alpha-lipoic acid, vitamin C.
7. **To improve insulin production and efficiency:** Chromium, biotin, zinc, magnesium, alpha-lipoic acid, bitter melon.

8. **To reduce stress:** Kava kava, vitamin C, Vitamin B₅ (pantothenic acid).

9. **To reduce inflammation and elevated CRP levels:** Systemic oral enzymes, Wobenzyme N, bromelain, MSM (methylsulfonylmethane).

10. **To build collagen for strong arteries:** Vitamin C, l-lysine, l-proline, MSM, copper, vitamin B₆, Aminogen.

11. **To reduce arterial plaque:** Niacin (as nicotinic acid), l-lysine, l-proline.

12. **To reduce and prevent free radical damage:** Alpha-lipoic acid, resveratrol, red grape extract, selenium, vitamin C, vitamin E, beta-carotene, mixed carotenes, l-gluthathione, green tea, astaxanthin, lycopene, chlorophyll, spirulina, soy.

13. **To lower blood pressure:** Potassium, magnesium, garlic (aged extract), l-arginine, EFAs.

14. **To improve blood circulation:** Ginkgo, EFAs, vitamin E, cayenne, garlic.

15. **To prevent blood clotting:** Resveratrol, vitamin K, EFAs, ginkgo.

16. **To lower cholesterol levels:** Niacin (as no-flush inositol hexaniacinate), artichoke extract, guggulipid, phytosterols, red yeast rice, garlic (aged extract), soy, alpha-lipoic acid.

17. **To oxygenate the blood:** Chlorophyll, copper, spirulina.

18. **To reduce excess weight:** Chromium, vanadium, EFAs, l-carnitine, biotin, bitter melon, bitter orange.

19. **To prevent against the damaging effects of dental infections/bacteria, smoking, alcohol, drugs:** Garlic, co-enzyme Q10, vitamin C, vitamin E, beta-carotene, selenium, folic acid, alpha-lipoic acid, resveratrol, red grape extract, vitamin C, mixed carotenes, l-gluthathione, green tea, astaxanthin, lycopene, chlorophyll, spirulina, soy.

Supplements for Optimum Cardiac Health

Consider the following dietary supplements to promote a healthy heart.

Alpha-Lipoic (Thioctic) Acid

One of the newer supplements to emerge on the dietary supplement scene, this superb bionutrient was first discussed by Snell, Thatum, and Peterson in the *Journal of Bacteria* back in 1937. In 1951, it attracted the serious interest of scientists. Dr. Lester Packer of the University of California at Berkeley pioneered alpha-lipoic acid research.

Alpha-lipoic acid, also referred to as lipoic acid, is a co-enzyme, a helper substance. Here is perhaps one of the most unique, protective, and beneficial nutrients for the cardiovascular system and whole body. To begin with, it is both a water-soluble and fat-soluble nutrient that is easily absorbed and very bioavailable, which means it can reach everywhere in the body, unlike nutrients that are only water or fat soluble. This water/fat-soluble substance is an aggressive antioxidant, blood sugar balancer, and chelating agent.

Lipoic acid quenches free radicals, particularly by neutralizing hydroxyl, hypochlorous, superoxide, peroxyl, and singlet oxygen free radicals. It interacts with and supports other antioxidants, helping to regenerate them, especially regenerating the antioxidant vitamins C and E. In 1959, Drs. Culik and Rosenberg demonstrated that alpha-lipoic acid prevents scurvy in vitamin C–deficient animals.

Alpha-lipoic acid improves glucose utilization and slows down the production of glucose. At high levels, 500 to 600 mg per day, lipoic acid increases glucose uptake and therefore lowers blood sugar. In diabetics, proteins tend to bind with sugar, which causes oxidative damage. Lipoic acid powerfully reduces the glycation (binding) of proteins with glucose. Its strong antioxidant activity thwarts the dangerous free radical damage caused by excess insulin circulating through the blood and excessive fat metabolism.

It is also a powerful chelating (binding) agent capable of binding with minerals in arterial plaques, especially toxic metals like lead, mercury, and cadmium. It readies them for excretion and removes them from artery walls and readies them for excretion. It regenerates gluthathione, its partner antioxidant, and lowers serum cholesterol. According to Dr. Richard Passwater, lipoic acid is a co-enzyme involved in the energy process, where it helps to liberate energy that the body forms as adenosine triphosphate (ATP).[1] Alpha-lipoic acid also neutralizes the effects of toxic metals that can damage mitochondria of cells.[2] Dr. Lester Packer's comments in a 1995 issue of *Free Radical Biology and Medicine* indicate that it protects against cholesterol oxidation and atherosclerosis in people with cardiovascular risk.[3]

Our Recommended Daily Amount: 200 mg for prevention; 200 to 400 mg for cardiovascular disease; 400 to 600 mg to lower glucose levels.

Aminogen

This ingenious patented and trademarked plant enzyme has the remarkable health-promoting ability to liberate free-form amino acids from any dietary protein food, such as soy, legumes, fish, poultry, and beef, whether it be of animal or plant origin. It dynamically multiplies the amounts of free-form amino acids that are released and become bioavailable from all protein foods. The Aminogen enzyme system breaks down and releases significantly more free-form amino acids from food than naturally secreted digestive enzymes alone. As a matter of fact, just 250 mg of Aminogen can release over 40,000 mg of amino acids!

As a sports supplement, Aminogen releases glutamine, which regulates body weight and composition. It also releases the BCAAs (branched-chain amino acids) isoleucine, leucine, and valine that promote protein synthesis, provide muscle fuel, combat fatigue, and strengthen the immune system. Arginine, a precursor to creatine and lysine that releases growth hormones, is also released in substantial amounts. Aminogen is also superb for children with increased amino acid needs.

Aminogen will also release higher amounts of lysine and proline, amino acids discussed earlier as the major components of hydroxy-proline and hydroxylysine, the precursors to collagen. As we get older, the body produces less digestive enzymes, creating conditions of achlorhydria (lack of stomach acid) and hypochlorhydria (low stomach acid production). With fewer digestive enzymes being produced by the pancreas, fewer free-form amino acids become available to the cells. Consequently, less lysine and proline are available to form collagen, required for arterial integrity and health. Small amounts of Aminogen can easily correct this problem.

Our Recommended Daily Amount: 250 mg with each meal.

Artichoke Extract (*Cynara scolymus*)

Derived from the common artichoke, this supplement has been historically used as a liver tonic and digestive aid. Artichoke is a choleretic, meaning that it stimulates the formation and flow of bile in the bile duct. Bile is a natural, yellowish, thick emulsifying fluid excreted from the liver and stored in the gallbladder, which assists the breakdown and absorption of fats as well as the breakdown of cholesterol in the small intestine.[4] Poor bile production causes malabsorption of fats and cholesterol. Artichoke extract efficiently metabolizes cholesterol. Its active ingredients, called caffeeylquinic acids, have the ability to turn down cholesterol production in the liver.[5] Recent findings reported in *PhytoMedicine* explain that artichoke also converts cholesterol to bile acids.[6] It is possible that some people have high cholesterol levels because they cannot convert cholesterol to bile acids. One study of more than five hundred people demonstrated that artichoke extract significantly lowered cholesterol levels.

Our Recommended Daily Amount: 120 to 360 mg, three times daily, of standardized extract of caffeylquinic acids.

Astaxanthin

This pink-colored phytonutrient appears to be one of the most powerful and promising antioxidants, a rising star in free radical scavenging ability and a welcome antioxidant to delicate eye tissues that are easily susceptible to oxidative damage. Recently emerging onto the natural products scene, natural astaxanthin is the plant pigment in ocean microalgae that gives crustaceans and salmon their pink color. One recent study demonstrated that natural source astaxanthin had more free radical scavenging power than synthetic astaxanthin, synthetic alpha-tocopherol, tocopherol, synthetic beta-carotene, lutein, and lycopene.

Our Recommended Daily Amount: follow directions on Supplement Facts panel.

Beta-Carotene/Carotenes

This well-studied group of over six hundred naturally occurring carotenes includes beta-carotene, alpha-carotene, lycopene, beta-cryptoxanthin, zeaxzathin, and cryptoxanthin—potent free radical–scavenging antioxidants. One study conducted by Dexter L. Morris, Ph.D., M.D., at the School of Medicine, University of North Carolina, Chapel Hill, cited that coronary artery disease can be prevented in part by the activity of mixed carotenoids in the blood, not just beta-carotene.[7]

A recent study published in *Annals of Epidemiology* reviewed findings from the National Health and Nutrition Examination Survey III (NANES III). E. S. Ford and colleagues analyzed the data and found that carotenoids in the blood were associated with a significantly lower risk of angina. They concluded that it made sense to take a group of mixed carotenoids resembling a more natural profile found in fruits and vegetables rather than just one type of carotenoid.[8]

Most important was the ability of carotenes to prevent oxidation of LDL (low-density lipoprotein) cholesterol. O. M. Panasenko and V. S. Sharov reported in their 2000 study that carotenes act as very powerful antioxidants against one of the most dangerous free radicals, peroxynitrite, a disease-promoting free radical composed of both oxygen and nitrogen atoms. Beta-carotene, alpha-carotene, and lycopene aggressively and effectively quenched peroxynitrite radicals in human LDL cholesterol before it became oxidized and contributory to the atherosclerotic process.[9]

Our Recommended Daily Amount: 15,000 IU (international units).

B-Complex

In addition to dozens of other essential functions, vitamins B_6, B_{12}, and folic acid reduce and eliminate homocysteine from the blood via the metabolic processes of methylation, remethylation, and transsulfuration. Research points out that the lowest levels of homocysteine in the blood are associated with the lowest risk of cardiovascular disease and conversely, the highest levels of homocysteine are associated with the highest risk. By constantly changing homocysteine back to methionine or converting it to harmless cysthathionine and clearing it from the blood, we dramatically reduce the cardiovascular risk and cardio destruction that too much homocysteine can cause. And basic vitamins, like B_6, inhibit platelet aggregation. This was known as far back as 1980, as explained in a study by A. Lam and colleagues.[10] A more recent study reported in the German journal *Arnzeim Forch* supported Lam's earlier findings that simple B_6 could effectively reduce a serious cardiovascular risk factor.[11]

Our Recommended Daily Amount: 50 to 100 mg B-complex.

Biotin

A B-complex vitamin, biotin is essential for the metabolism of fats, carbohydrates, and proteins. It is not considered an essential vitamin, since we can make it with the help of bacteria in the digestive tract. Interestingly, biotin is probably the most underutilized and poorly studied dietary supplement for the management of diabetes. Yet it has a major function in the control of blood sugar and should be on everyone's list for glucose regulation, especially for diabetics or anyone with blood sugar disorders.

Biotin increases insulin sensitivity and enhances the activity of glucokinase, the enzyme critical to the efficient first step in the utilization of sugar by the liver.[12] This was the conclusion presented by A. Reddi and colleagues in a 1988 *Life Sciences* paper. Typical biotin levels in diabetics are low. Therapeutic blood sugar balancing and stabilizing effects of biotin have been reported at 9 mg (9,000 mcg) per day. Because it is a water-soluble B-complex vitamin, there is no known danger or toxicity associated with massive doses. In the future, biotin will appear in more supplements for diabetics combined with other nutrients. When beginning supplementation with biotin, it is advisable to speak to your doctor if you are diabetic, as it will likely lower your insulin requirements.

Our Recommended Daily Amount: for prevention—500 mcg; for blood sugar regulation and diabetic therapy—7,000 to 9,000 mcg.

Bitter Melon (*Momordica charantia*)

This is a green, bumpy, cucumber-shaped tropical fruit native to Asia, Africa, and South America. The fresh juice of this unripe fruit contains well-documented antidiabetic properties. Bitter melon boosts pancreatic beta cell activity and may lower plasma glucose levels. Charantin, the primary active substance in bitter melon, is a powerful hypoglycemic composed of mixed plant steroids that studies show possess greater efficacy than prescription drugs like tolbutamide.

Bitter melon also contains polypeptide P, an insulin-like substance that lowers blood sugar levels in Type I diabetics. It is an effective blood sugar–lowering substance.[13] Bitter melon does not interfere with prescription medications, but initiates a hypoglycemic effect that requires daily monitoring.

Our Recommended Daily Amount: 100 to 200 mg.

Bitter Orange (*Citrus aurantium*)

Commonly known as bitter orange, this ancient Chinese herb called *Zhi shi* is a new, thermogenic alternative and healthy, natural approach to weight loss. It is the ideal replacement for ephedra (*Ma huang*) as a powerful thermogenic (heat-creating) and lipolytic (fat breakdown) ingredient. Bitter orange is similar in action to ephedra, but does not have the same potential for producing cardiovascular and nervous system side effects when used at the appropriate dosage. Standardized extracts of 6 percent *citrus aurantium*, plus a natural composition of five adrenergic amines (organic compounds from plants able to release or behave as stress hormones adrenaline and noradrenaline) appear to switch metabolism into a fat-burning rather than a carbohydrate-burning mode. Bitter orange also accelerates the metabolic rate to burn calories much faster.

Our Recommended Daily Amount: Follow directions on Supplement Facts panel.

Cayenne (*Capsicum frutescens*)

Native to tropical America and one of the most familiar and widely used condiments in the world, cayenne is the fruit (berry) of the plant. Containing the active ingredient capsaicin, which also gives it its zesty and irritating properties, cayenne boosts the metabolic rate and increases blood flow to peripheral areas. It has antioxidant properties because of its carotene content.

Cayenne lowers triglycerides and cholesterol while reducing platelet aggregation and clotting activity in much the same way as garlic.[14,15] In populations where the consumption of cayenne is high, cardiovascular disease rates are lower. Of special interest is its ability to increase circulation, particularly peripheral genital circulation, effectively reducing erectile dysfunction. Cayenne can be consumed freely in food.

Our Recommended Daily Amount: 100 mg, three times daily.

Chlorophyll

Few single nutrients on the planet can be compared to the nutritional uniqueness and life-giving benefits of chlorophyll, the green pigment found in all green foods (fruits, vegetables, cereal grasses, spirulina, blue-green algae, all green land plants, seaweeds, and green food supplements). Chlorophyll is at the center of a unique natural process called photosynthesis that occurs continuously within green life. You might vaguely remember from high school biology class that photosynthesis is a complex and not thoroughly understood chemical process. This process uses the chlorophyll molecules present in plants to collect energy found in and given off by natural sunlight streaming down toward earth. Once it is captured, the energy in sunlight is converted via many complex and not totally understandable steps to chemical energy. Once produced, this chemical energy is harnessed and put to work by the plant. It converts the water it draws from the soil and carbon dioxide from the air into easily and readily accessible food energy in the forms of simple sugars, carbohydrates, proteins, and the oxygen needed to 'burn" the food energy. No other single substance on earth can make that claim!

Chlorophyll, of which there are several types, belongs to a special group of biologically vital substances found in the body. Hemoglobin (the body's oxygen-transporting protein in the blood), myoglobin (the body's oxygen storage protein in muscle), and cytochrome (an oxygen storage and transfer protein) are interestingly all members of this group. From a chemical point of view, chlorophyll, hemoglobin, myoglobin, and cytochrome are very similar. All have chemical structures that are nearly identical, with each containing a protein called globin. The center of each molecule, however, is different. Hemoglobin has iron at its center, surrounded by globin. It is the molecule that facilitates cellular respiration, by picking up oxygen from the lungs and carrying it in the bloodstream to cells throughout the body. Chlorophyll has magnesium at its center with globin around it and is also believed to transport oxygen.

Chlorophyll exerts powerful maintenance, protective, and therapeutic effects within the body. Perhaps chlorophyll's most important role is played as a highly efficient tune-up, clean-up, and detoxifying agent for the liver, our primary chemical factory, keeping it running in top form. Chlorophyll stimulates the production of hemoglobin, protein that transports oxygen to cells, especially heart muscle cells. When the liver receives sufficient oxygen on a regular basis, it is able to manufacture specialized enzymes, particularly the cytochrome P450 complex. This highly specialized enzyme group neutralizes toxins efficiently and quickly, and then makes them water soluble for easy elimination. This prevents extremely reactive free radicals from accumulating and causing future damage to arterial tissues and in the liver.[16,17]

As far back as 1855, scientist Verdel proposed the nearly identical nature of chlorophyll and hemoglobin. The theory that chlorophyll and hemoglobin are interchangeable in the oxygen transport process is somewhat reasonable, yet it is not conclusive. However, a more accurate and acceptable theory, supported by scientific evidence and anecdotal reports, states that greens stimulate the production of hemoglobin in the blood. As a result, a higher concentration of oxygen circulating through the arteries is available, waiting to be plucked out by oxygen-hungry cells, particularly in heart muscle.

To a limited extent, the idea that chlorophyll mimics the oxygen-carrying activity of hemoglobin is accurate. A study in 1970 by Hammel-Dupont and Bessman, reported in *Biochemical Medicine*, conveyed the idea that chlorophyll stimulated and facilitated reproduction of the globin (protein) portion of hemoglobin. The globin molecule was then capable of picking up an iron molecule, becoming a molecule of hemoglobin. An increased quantity of hemoglobin molecules in the blood means more oxygen pickup in the lungs, more oxygen-carrying capacity, and consequently, more oxygen-rich blood for transport to cells for use as metabolic energy.

Our Recommended Daily Amount: 50 to 100 mg.

Chromium

Suspected as a necessary dietary mineral in the 1950s, this trace micro-mineral is essential for insulin formation in the pancreas. Whole grains, legumes, and brewer's yeast are rich dietary sources. Vital for balanced sugar metabolism, chromium enables insulin to bind to receptors so that sugar can enter the cell. It controls appetite, cravings for food, and desire for sweets. Chromium also increases the ability of insulin receptors that help the eye muscle focus. The signs of chromium deficiency include: fasting hyperglycemia, impaired glucose tolerance, hyperinsulinemia, decreased insulin receptors, decreased insulin binding, and elevated body fat.

Studies and investigations show that most people are deficient in chromium, with the average intake for self-directed diets at about 35 mcg for men and 25 mcg for women.[18] This is well below the DV (Daily Value) of 120 mcg and far below 200 to 290 mcg, which is considered optimum for healthy people. Obviously, supplementation is strongly recommended.

Chromium lowers fasting glucose levels and increases the number of insulin receptors in adipocytes (fat cells), muscle, and liver. In addition, it boosts the binding activity of insulin to its receptors and multiplies the number of insulin receptors on cells.[19] Chromium also regulates enzymes at the cellular level to increase phosphate-group binding to cells. More phosphate groups mean greater sensitivity to insulin, increasing its efficiency. Chromium is also capable of inhibiting an enzyme called tyrosine phosphatase, responsible for terminating the insulin receptor response. Its dual action of increasing glucose binding and negating the binding termination response makes chromium an effective controller of glucose utilization.

A 1997 issue of *Diabetes* published a study by R. A. Anderson and colleagues at the USDA (United States Department of Agriculture) showing the effects of chromium supplementation on Type II diabetics. Those people in the study who took large doses of chromium for several months experienced a lowering of glucose and insulin in their blood back to levels that were almost normal.[20] Other studies demonstrated that triglycerides could be lowered with chromium supplementation, offering protection against cardiovascular disease.[21] A 1980 issue of *Diabetes* reported that chromium in the form of chromium polynicotinate (chromium with the nicotinic acid form of niacin), referred to in the literature as glucose tolerance factor (GTF chromium), was considered an effective and safe form of chromium for dietary supplementation.[22] Research studies show that niacin-bound chromium is more readily absorbed than other forms and is very effective at promoting normal levels of blood sugar, cholesterol, and triglycerides, while increasing energy. Glucose tolerance factor niacin bound chromium and chelated chromium (chromium bound to an amino acid) are effective sources. Chromium is extremely safe, and no toxicity level is known.

Our Recommended Daily Amount: for prevention—200 mcg as glucose tolerance factor (GTF) chromium. For diabetes and other blood sugar disorders—200 mcg three times daily and *advise your physician.*

Co-Enzyme A

Discovered in 1947, co-enzyme A is a metabolic enzyme manufactured in the liver that operates in the body's cells and blood. It initiates the Krebs cycle, which is responsible for producing about 95 percent of the body's energy needed to sustain life. This cycle, which initiates fatty acid, carbohydrate, and protein metabolism, is involved in the production of energy and the transport of fats to and from cells. Co-enzyme A also initiates the metabolic cycle responsible for breaking down sugar. Pantethine, a form of the essential B vitamin pantothenic acid, is the most important component of co-enzyme A. It also initiates the production of hormones, especially cortisol, which controls blood sugar levels and stress. Co-enzyme A can be made in the body from ATP (adenosine triphosphate), the amino acid cysteine, and vitamin B_5 (pantothenic acid). We can manufacture ATP and cysteine, but we must get B_5 from our diet.

Our Recommended Daily Amount: follow directions on Supplement Facts panel.

Co-Enzyme Q10 (Ubiquinone)

This unique fat-soluble, vitamin-like nutrient, obtained from food and synthesized by the body in small amounts, is an essential part of the body's energy-producing system. First identified in the 1940s, co-enzyme Q10 (CoQ10) is chemically similar to vitamin K. It does its work in the inner mitochondrial membrane, assisting in the production of ATP and the utilization of energy. Co-enzyme Q10 works in every cell of the body as an antioxidant and maintains cell membranes. Co-enzyme Q10 also improves postsurgical recovery if taken in advance of heart surgery. In a 1993 study reported by *Clinical Investigator*, congestive heart failure patients exhibited significant changes—positive improvements in cardiac function—when taking co-enzyme Q10.[23] According to Karl Folkers, a prominent co-enzyme Q10 researcher, CoQ10 improves the symptoms of heart failure and angina.[24]

Co-enzyme Q10 is a critical nutrient for people with cardiovascular problems who typically take some form of medication to reduce or eliminate symptoms. One major concern is that cholesterol-lowering drugs, such as Zocor and Mevacor, while trying to lower cholesterol, actually deplete vital CoQ10 stores in the blood and heart.

Our Recommended Daily Amount: 50 mg is recommended for prevention; 100 to 200 mg for therapeutic use.

Copper

This essential mineral, found in shellfish, nuts, seeds, cocoa powder, and legumes, has many functions. For the heart and cardiovascular system it is essential for proper cross-linking of collagen. Copper is part of many enzyme complexes, especially the enzyme lysyl oxidase, which acts on lysine and proline components of collagen to help form strong cross-links of collagen and build connective tissue in the arteries and other tissues. Copper is an integral part of cytochrome P oxidase, considered a critical enzyme in humans to help form ATP, our primary energy molecule. It also helps transport iron in hemoglobin. Copper is a part of SOD (superoxide dismutase), which is a major free radical–scavenging antioxidant in the liver.

Our Recommended Daily Amount: 1.5 to 3 mg.

D-Ribose

One of the newest entries into the ever-growing nutritional supplement arsenal, this polysaccharide (complex sugar), is present in every cell of the body. It is also found in many foods. Unknown to most of us and to many health professionals as well, this silent nutritional powerhouse was discussed by H. G. Segal and H. Foley in 1958 in their journal paper, "The Metabolism of D-Ribose in Man." D-ribose is responsible for starting the metabolic process that generates ATP (adenosine triphosphate), the body's primary energy molecule, in all living cells. D-ribose also accelerates the recycling of ATP. This supports healthy cardiovascular function and the function of skeletal muscle tissues.[25]

In order for muscles to function, they need this energy in the form of ATP. It is what allows muscles to do work, whether it is walking, lifting, breathing, or most important, the beating of your heart. When excessive demands are placed on muscles by exercise, oxygen levels decrease. As a result, the demand for ATP rises dramatically, but the body can't keep up. Muscle levels of ATP are drained, particularly in the heart. Your body can lose 60 to 70 percent of its ATP supply after long, exhausting exercise, and it can take more than seventy-two hours for it to be restored.[26] Obviously, energy, endurance, and strength are poor during this period and why this happens is simple. During periods of intense activity or oxygen depletion, our muscles lose building-block molecules called adenine nucleotides (ANs) because they leak into the bloodstream through the cell membranes. Our muscles cannot regenerate and replace ATP without first restoring ANs. This characteristically slow process in heart and skeletal muscle is due to an insufficient amount of glucose 6-phosphate dehydrogenase (an enzyme) needed in the AN synthesis pathway. This imposes a limit to the rate at which ANs and ATP can form again.[27] Here's where the uniqueness of d-ribose comes into play. It can skip past the rate-limiting enzyme-dependent process. Then it forms ANs as soon as it enters the cell.[28] This unique ability was reported by E. Zimmer and colleagues in the *Journal of Molecular Cell Cardiology* in 1984. Because d-ribose is so safe, dozens of research studies conducted both on healthy and unhealthy humans show that practically everyone can benefit from its use.

Of special interest is the use of d-ribose for cardiac health and recovery. The 1992 study by Pliml tested and monitored patients with coronary artery disease after exercise-induced ischemia (oxygen deprivation). The study group of ten was given d-ribose for three days. All ten significantly increased their exercise time—a 30 percent improvement in pain-free exercise time compared to no improvement, and a 50 percent decline in exercise time in the placebo group. Interestingly, two patents have been issued for d-ribose use in open-heart surgery. Finally, in a comprehensive university study by Gross in 1989, the highlights of d-ribose use were summarized, citing that it is well tolerated in amounts up to 14 grams for a 150-pound man. Its peak concentration in blood is reached in one to two hours. Ninety-five percent of d-ribose is absorbed into the bloodstream. It does not change blood pressure, heart rate, or blood values. And d-ribose has a blood sugar–lowering effect.

Our Recommended Daily Amount: for a healthy heart and muscles, 8 grams twice daily, one hour before exercise and thirty minutes before bed.

EFAs (Essential Fatty Acids)

Omega-3 EFAs are found in flax seeds, walnuts, salmon, mackerel, sardines, and other cold-water fish. Omega-6 EFAs, found in nut and seed meats and their oils, such as almond, canola, corn, sesame, sunflower, safflower, flax, and soybean, provide countless nutritional benefits that power critical metabolic functions, maintain biological integrity, and promote homeostasis (balance). They keep cell membranes soft, elastic, and pliable.

Omega-3 EFAs lower blood pressure throughout the body's arterial network and reduce LDL cholesterol. Omega-3 derivatives prevent dangerous blood clotting, reduce inflammation, and support healthy brain function. GLA (gamma linolenic acid), an omega-6 EFA derivative, is not officially essential because we can make it internally, but it is regarded by many health experts to be essential for optimal wellness. GLA is abundant in borage, evening primrose, and black currant oils. GLA shrinks prostate and systemic inflammation by converting to anti-inflammatory localized hormonelike substances called prostaglandins.

Our Recommended Daily Amount: 300 to 600 mg.

Flax

Few foods can compare in nutritional value to flax. It is an ancient plant with a recorded use in history that dates to the old Egyptian civilizations. Europeans and Native Americans used flax for hundreds of years before the Industrial Age. Many of those cultures harvested and pressed fresh oil from flax seeds. Native American Cherokees believed that flax captured the sun's energy to be used in the body. Noted German doctor JoAnna Budwig has spent a lifetime researching flax and its therapeutic uses. Her flax oil and protein regimen is known and highly regarded worldwide.

Flax is the richest source of omega-3 fats on the planet, containing nearly 60 percent omega-3s. Flax is also rich in omega-6 fats, about 18 percent, plus beta-carotene and vitamin E. It has more omega-3s than fish because the omega-3 EFAs in fish come from the green microalgae and ocean vegetation that the fish eat. Among its many benefits: flax improves oxygenation of the blood and cells; reduces vascular and systemic inflammation; and lowers blood pressure, cholesterol, and triglycerides.[30]

Omega-3s in flax are precursors to prostaglandins that reduce inflammation. An old but valuable study conducted in 1964, published in *The Lancet*, revealed that omega-3 from flax reduced the stickiness of platelets. Many studies support the premise that omega-3s have powerful antioxidant properties.

Our Recommended Daily Amount: A minimum of .16 gram per pound of body weight of combined omega-3 and omega-6 EFAs. This is approximately 24 grams of EFAs for a 150-pound person. Healthy suggested ratios are 10:1 to 4:1 and 4:1 to 1:1, omega-6 to omega-3. We recommend getting 5 to 10 grams of omega-3s and 10 to 20 of grams omega-6s per day, from foods or supplements.

Folic Acid

Levels of homocysteine in the blood are carefully controlled by a combination of nutritional and genetic factors, among which is the enzyme methylenetetrahydrofolate reductase (MTHFR). A defective variation of this enzyme is clearly associated with elevated homocysteine. Increased blood plasma levels of homocysteine are directly correlated to a genetic inheritance of this defective enzyme. In the November 1996 issue of *Circulation*, Gallagher, Meleady, and their researchers at the Department of Genetics, Trinity College, Dublin, Ireland, reported that the presence of the defective MTHFR enzyme apparently increased the risk of premature coronary artery disease. They concluded that genetically correct MTHFR, which effectively controls the homocysteine concentration in the blood, is totally dependent on folate, and that supplementation may reduce the risk.

Each year more than twelve million people die as a result of various cardiovascular diseases, particularly from heart attacks and strokes. The 1998 E. B. Rimm–W. C. Willet study published in the *Journal of the American Medical Association* established the relationship and importance of folate and vitamin B_6 in the prevention of cardiovascular disease.[31] Lane Leonhard, Ph.D., in his September 1998 *Vitamin Research News*, reviewed the 1995 Boushey study that was published in the *Journal of the American Medical Association*. Dr. Leohnard suggested that 13,500 to 50,000 deaths from cardiovascular disease could be prevented by including about twenty-five cent's worth of B vitamins per day in the diet.[32]

The scientific information suggesting that lowering the risk of heart disease, sudden death, and early mortality by supplementing with folic acid is very convincing. A revealing study featured in the January 1998 issue of *The Lancet* examined thirty-eight patients with a combination of progressive atherosclerosis of the carotid artery and high homocysteine levels. During an eighteen-month trial period, the group was given supplemental folic acid, B_6, and B_{12}. The promising result was that arterial lesions stopped progressing and regressed slightly, suggesting that similar results could be achieved in larger population studies.

Another eye-opening study conducted by R. M. Russell in 1996 was published in the *Journal of the American Medical Association*. It stated that a minimum of 13,500 deaths from coronary artery disease could be prevented each year by simply increasing the intake of folic acid to lower homocysteine levels in the blood.[33] Furthermore, another, newer study published in the November 1998 *Annals of Epidemiology*, conducted by Giles-Kittner and team, examined the relationship of folate and the risk for coronary heart disease. The results, compiled from a group of U.S. adults and collected by the First National Health and Nutrition Examination Survey Epidemiologic Follow-Up Study, put forth the hypothesis that risk factors for heart disease related to a lack of folic acid were age related and that risk increased with age.

Our Recommended Daily Amount: 400 mcg for cardiovascular health, 800 mcg for therapeutic use in cardiovascular disease, and 1,200 mcg to lower homocysteine.

Garlic (*Allium sativum*)

One of civilization's oldest natural health remedies with thousands of years of documented use, this member of the lily family is cultivated worldwide. Its use was recorded in Sanskrit over five thousand years ago and it has been part of the Chinese culinary and medicinal culture for more than three thousand years. *Codex Ebers*, a medical papyrus from Egypt, records the use of garlic for medicinal purposes including hypertension. Garlic was also written about on cuneiform tablets in 3,000 B.C. These tablets document that the ancient Sumerians and Assyrians used garlic for a variety of medicinal purposes as well. Hippocrates also mentioned garlic for its therapeutic medicinal benefits. A concoction of macerated garlic and wine was used in France during the early 1700s to give immunity from disease. The natural healing power of garlic has endured for thousands of years.

The bulb, often referred to the "stinking rose," contains several reportedly beneficial medicinal substances. Garlic contains a volatile oil composed of allicin and sulfur compounds, such as diallyl sulfide, S-allylcysteine, and gammaglutamylpeptides, alliin, alliinase, diallyltrisulfide, s-allyl-l-cysteine sulfoxide, plus high levels of antioxidant selenium. Regular consumption of garlic can protect against heart attacks and strokes. Many studies show that numerous components of garlic, derived from fresh garlic bulbs, garlic powder, and aged garlic extracts, effectively reduce LDL cholesterol levels, raise HDL cholesterol, lower triglycerides, and lower blood pressure.

This nutritional wonder reduces platelet adhesiveness and increases clotting activity, which can decrease the risk of atherosclerotic disease.[34] One of garlic's most valuable activities is its ability to prevent the oxidation of LDL cholesterol. In 1993 A. Phelps and K. Arris demonstrated the ability of garlic to reduce exposure of LDL cholesterol to oxidation. And in 1999, a study conducted by N. Ide and B. H. S. Lau at Loma Linda University in California described the ability of s-allyl cysteine, a component of aged garlic extract, to exert potent antioxidant activity to prevent oxidation of LDL.[35] A second study by the same research team also confirmed that another component of aged garlic extract, fructosyl arginine, contributes to the antioxidant effects on LDLs.[36] Because active components relax blood vessels, garlic lowers blood pressure.[37]

Garlic, also renowned for its aggressive antibacterial, antifungal, antiparasitic, and immune system–stimulating activity and abilities, is a powerful bionutrient in the control of diabetes. In 1999, S. Kasuga and colleagues studied the risk of diabetes mellitus, hyperglycemia, and aged garlic extract. They demonstrated that aged garlic extract significantly prevented hyperglycemia, and its effectiveness was the same as for diazepam, a widely prescribed medication for the treatment of diabetes. They concluded that this garlic extract may prevent stress-induced hyperglycemia, which is the risk of suffering from diabetes mellitus and its progression.[38]

Another 1999 study by Ide and Lau examined the effects of aged garlic extract in connection with important atherosclerosis risk markers, such as free radical oxidation and destruction of LDL cholesterol within pulmonary artery cells. Aged garlic extract prevented injury to arterial cells caused by oxidation, primarily by protecting the depletion of gluthathione and eliminating toxins. We can conclude from this study that aged garlic extract is an effective nutritional weapon for preventing the development of atherosclerosis and cardiovascular diseases.[39] In the face of noxious, synthetic pharmaceutical drugs, we should pay more attention to the natural medicinal abilities of garlic. Let's take a lesson from the ancients!

Our Recommended Daily Amount: for maximum effect, 4 to 8 grams fresh garlic (1 to 2 medium to large cloves) or the prepared product equivalent.

Ginkgo (*Ginkgo biloba*)

Ginkgo biloba trees are the earth's oldest, often referred to as living fossils. They survived the Ice Age in China and were then elevated to sacred status. A time-honored, traditional Chinese medicine remedy, ginkgo is referred to as far back as 2,800 B.C. for providing brain and other medicinal benefits.[40] Ginkgo made its way to Europe in 1730 and is now used there extensively to improve mental ability and alertness.[41] Doctors in Germany write more prescriptions for ginkgo than any other natural medicine.

This favorite ancient tree supplies active leaf extract substances called ginkoflavonglycosides, ginkgolides, and terpene lactones. Ginkgo also stimulates peripheral circulation and blood supply, specifically in genitalia, to decrease erectile dysfunction symptoms. Ginkgo has the ability, unlike many other nutrients, to cross the blood-brain barrier to improve cerebral circulation. This raises oxygen levels, heightens memory, and prevents clotting in microcapillaries.[42] It reduces the incidence and formation of varicose veins. Ginkgo also contains antioxidants that battle free radicals and supports circulation in small vessels.

Our Recommended Daily Amount: a standardized extract of 24/6 percent ginkgoflavonglycosides and terpene lactones, 80 mg, three times daily.

Grapeseed Extract

The simple grape is home to many superpowerful antioxidants such as resveratrol, ellagic acid, and OPCs (oligomeric proanthocyanidins), or PCOs (proanthocyanidins), natural antioxidants with powerful pharmacological and biological protective properties. They are colorless until they interact with other plant nutrients, which turn them into anthocyanidins having a deep purple-blue or red color.

The first recorded use of these special substances occurred in 1534 when Jacques Cartier explored the Saint Lawrence River. When his crew developed signs of scurvy, a Native American told him to make pine-needle tea for them. Those who drank the tea survived. The active ingredients in grapeseed were originally discovered, identified, and isolated back in 1948 by the well-known French scientist Jacques Masquelier at the University of Bordeaux. What he found was a co-factor substance, OPC, that was capable of reducing the fragility of capillaries, preventing them from rupturing, improving blood and lymph vessel function throughout the body, and reducing swollen tissue.

In 1951, he patented the extraction method from Maritime pine bark, familiar as pycnogenol, and from grape seeds in 1970. Pine bark contains 80 to 85 percent PCOs and grapeseed contains 90 to 95 percent, making it a better source. OPCs protect us from free radical damage in the same way they protect the plant. OPCs inhibit the breakdown of vitamin C, increasing the duration of its effectiveness. A 1998 study in *General Pharmacology* stated that grapeseed OPCs have greater antioxidant effects than vitamin C and vitamin E.[43]

The main cardiovascular benefit of OPCs is quite important. Simply, they inhibit the destruction of collagen, the vital structure for connective tissues, particularly the arteries and blood vessels. PCOs accomplish this by cross-linking collagen fibers, which reinforces the natural cross-linking of the existing collagen matrix.[44] They prevent the oxidation of cholesterol and fats, avoiding formation of lipid peroxides and cholesterol epoxides. They also prevent the splitting up of collagen by enzymes that are sent out by leucocytes during inflammatory episodes.

Our Recommended Daily Amount: 75 mg for overall cardiovascular protection; 150 mg to correct health problems.

Green Tea (*Camellia sinensis*)

Green tea is the third most popular beverage in the world, behind coffee and black tea. Many people in this country don't really understand what it is. When tea leaves are harvested, one of several things happens. The leaves can be lightly steamed to stop the natural fermentation process, and this produces green tea. When the leaves are only partially fermented, it produces Oolong tea. And when the leaves are allowed to fully ferment, black tea is produced. Green tea, widely consumed in Asian countries, is a major factor responsible for lower cardiovascular disease rates in Japan than in America. Even though it is reported that more than 50 percent of Japanese men smoke and consume a high-salt diet, they have a lower rate of heart disease.

Green tea hosts a unique profile of phytonutrients, particularly a special polyphenol found in green tea, epigallocatechin gallate (EGCG). EGCG is the most powerful antioxidant in green tea and prevents lipid peroxidation.[45] Numerous studies point out that EGCG is capable of almost totally inhibiting free radical damage to LDL cholesterol.[46] Green tea has been shown in animal studies to keep cholesterol in normal range. And green tea does even more to control cholesterol, according to a 1992 study by I. Ikeda and colleagues. The study revealed that EGCG inhibited the absorption of cholesterol by hooking up with bile salts and emulsified cholesterol to form an insoluble substance that cannot be absorbed by the intestines and is excreted in feces.[47]

Green tea lowers blood pressure, too. In one study reported in a 1995 issue of the *Journal of Cardiovascular Pharmacology*, it was ranked fifth out of fifty-four plant foods shown to relax the endothelial blood vessel lining, and it produced a 91 percent relaxation.[48] Green tea has been the subject of hundreds of scientific studies in the past decade. Many health experts consider it one of the ten most important foods to include in the diet.

The research of Dr. C. A. Rice-Evans of the Free Radical Research Group of Guys Hospital, London, published in 1996 in *Free Radical Biology and Medicine*, concluded that the flavonoids in green tea (in the catechin family) were more efficient antioxidants than their powerful counterparts beta-carotene, vitamin E, and vitamin C.[49] Finally, several studies reported in journals worldwide show that green tea prevents dangerous blood clotting because it keeps the blood less sticky and prevents the formation of the blood-clotting eicosanoid called thromboxane.[50]

Our Recommended Daily Amount: 100 mg, two times daily is recommended. Better yet, drink two to four mugs of green tea. *If you are sensitive to caffeine try decaffeinated versions.*

Guggulipid (*Commiphora mukul*)

Called gum Gugul or guggulu, this is a yellowish tree gum resin derived from the root of the short, thorny, mukhul myrhh tree, native to India and Asia. This is a key botanical medicine used in ancient Ayurveda, the traditional system of medicine practiced in India. It is described in the classic medicine text, *Sushrusamhita*, for obesity treatment, fat disorders, and "coating and obstruction of channels." In 600 B.C., Ayurvedic physicians diagnosed atherosclerosis (hardening of the arteries with plaques) and treated it with guggul.

The resin, which has a balsamic aroma, is split up for medical use. Its neutral portion, which contains the unique phytonutrients Z and

E guggulsterones, demonstrates the ability to lower LDL and VLDL (very low density lipoprotein) cholesterol, total serum lipids, and triglycerides, and raises HDL.[51] The mechanism of action is clear. Guggulipid actually lowers cholesterol by increasing the liver's metabolism of LDL cholesterol.[52]

To date guggulipid has not exhibited any negative side effects in clinical studies. It does not adversely affect kidney function, blood sugar control, liver function, or hematological (blood serum) parameters. It is safe during pregnancy, with no fetotoxic (toxic to the fetus) or embryotoxic (toxic to the embryo) effects having been observed. The LD 50 (50 percent toxic dose) is approximately 727 mg per pound of body weight; in other words, over one hundred capsules per day. This is very safe! The cholesterol-and triglyceride-lowering power of guggulipid is comparable to that of drugs which lower cholesterol and lipids, without the side effects. Guggul also exerts strong anti-inflammatory action.

Our Recommended Daily Amount: standardized extract containing 25 mg guggulsterones, three times daily.

Hawthorn (*Crataegus oxyacantha*)

This spiny shrublike tree, native to Europe, produces berries, leaves, and blossoms with extremely heart-healthy medicinal benefits. Hawthorn holds a key component of heart health. It contains antioxidant phytonutrient flavonoids, especially anthocyanidins and proanthocyanidins that give it the red-blue colors also found in blueberries, blackberries, cherries, and other fruits. Hawthorn flowers contain quercetin and the active phytonutrient vitexin. Hawthorn is also rich in cardiotonic amines that strengthen the heart's action.[53]

Traditionally used as a tonic for angina, congestive heart failure, high blood pressure, and atherosclerosis, hawthorn berries improve the overall efficiency of the heart. Hawthorn also has the ability to naturally dilate coronary arteries by relaxing smooth muscle. It accomplishes this by downregulating the activity of angiotensin-converting enzyme, which converts angiotensin I (a powerful vasoconstricting enzyme) to angiotensin II (a mild vasoconstricting enzyme). This action enlarges the opening of the artery and improves blood supply by allowing more blood to flow.

The phytonutrients in hawthorn improve the overall metabolic processes of the heart in two interesting ways. First, they increase the force of contraction of the heart muscle, which in turn increases the amount of blood flow per beat, known medically as the ejection fraction. Second, hawthorn smoothes out rhythm disturbances that can occur in the heart's electrical cycle.[54] Of particular interest is that the flavonoids in hawthorn have powerful collagen-stabilizing action. This prevents dangerous breakdown of the fibrous structure of collagen that is essential to the integrity and strength of your arteries. The stabilization process is accomplished by cross-linking collagen fibers to form a sturdy matrix. And by virtue of the stabilization process, hawthorn prevents susceptibility to arterial injury.[55]

Hawthorn is also a powerful antioxidant capable of preventing free radical damage. Hawthorn has been shown to improve oxygen utilization, too. And it reduces cholesterol and atherosclerotic plaques by stabilizing collagen, thereby protecting it from free radical damage while decreasing capillary fragility and permeability.[56] Hawthorn can also inhibit the release and synthesis of substances that promote inflammation such as leukotrienes, histamine, and prostaglandins that can inflame arteries. Other species (*c. monogyna* and *c. pentagyna*) exert similar pharmacological activity and are acceptable substitutes for preventive and therapeutic use. Concentrated amounts of procyanidins and vitexin increase the efficiency of the heart. They improve the blood and oxygen supply by dilating coronary vessels and increasing blood-pumping capacity, while decreasing resistance of blood vessels. Hawthorn renders the heart stronger, healthier, and more efficient.[57,58]

Our Recommended Daily Amount: 150 to 250 mg standardized extract (1.8 percent vitexin), three times daily.

Kava kava (*Piper methysticum*)

The kavalactones in this ancient Polynesian "feel good" herb will safely take the edge off practically everyone's stress. This South Pacific shrub has been keeping the natives calm for thousands of years. Fresh or dried roots yield calming, antianxiety kavalactones. While kava kava is no substitute for good stress reduction techniques and lifestyle changes, it will mellow you out when things get too hyper and out of control.

Our Recommended Daily Amount: a 30 percent or 55 percent kavalactones standardized extract yielding 45 to 70 mg, three times daily. *Not intended for use during pregnancy, lactation, or clinical depression.*

L-Arginine

A nonessential amino acid in adults but essential in children, arginine is a precursor to nitric oxide (also known as EDRF—endothelial relaxation factor), which acts as a vasodilator that lowers blood pressure. It relaxes arteries to prevent heart-stopping spasms or extreme injury that causes pressure on artery walls.[59,60] Arginine also increases blood flow, particularly peripheral blood flow to the extremities, which prevents the development of peripheral vascular disease.

For people who suffer from heart failure, taking arginine before exercise is the "Batman and Robin" dynamic duo. Arginine, naturally found in nuts, seeds, and meats, is a nutritional dynamo for healthy blood circulation. According to Mary Mayell, author of *Off the Shelf Natural Health* (Bantam Books, 1995), arginine, although not considered nutritionally essential, may be required by adults with specific health problems, above all, cardiovascular problems.

The first prospective randomized clinical trial of its kind, published in the *Journal of the American College of Cardiology*, concluded that arginine combined with exercise had an enhanced energizing effect on people with chronic heart failure who typically have a damaged endothelium. Their blood vessels don't expand naturally. Arginine, which dilates the vessels, allows for better blood flow.[61] A key symptom of chronic heart failure is exercise intolerance due to inadequate blood flow, so improving blood flow in these patients may limit muscle fatigue and result in better endurance. And many other l-arginine studies have shown that in people with high blood pressure or high cholesterol levels it has an artery-dilating effect.

Many men are concerned with their ability to maintain sexual function as they age. Arginine is a powerful preventive against impotence or reverser of existing impotence because it helps relax arteries in the penis, allowing for better blood flow to achieve and maintain an erection.

Some people should not take l-arginine: those who are predisposed to herpes outbreaks and cancer patients (arginine may increase the replication of the virus or replication of cancer cells). Arginine should also not be taken by people with low blood pressure and those with liver and kidney problems. Those taking blood thinners or hypotensive drugs should consult their doctors before taking arginine. It can trigger growth hormone activity, so it may burden the pancreas in some people. Pregnant women are also advised to avoid l-arginine supplements. People with chronic heart failure may take arginine under the supervision of a cardiologist. But for all others, arginine can safely lower blood pressure and increase blood flow.

Our Recommended Daily Amount: 500 mg, three times daily.

L-Carnitine

Originally isolated from beef in 1905, l-carnitine was chemically identified in 1927. The term *carnitine* comes from the Latin word *carnis*, meaning "flesh." This vitamin-like substance is a multipurpose workhorse for your cardiovascular system. It was demonstrated by I. B. Fritz in the 1950s to be essential for long-chain fatty acid metabolism in the heart and muscle.[62] L-carnitine plays a critical role in the conversion of fat to energy in the heart by efficiently accelerating the burning of fats for energy in the mitochondria (furnaces) of the heart cells.

L-carnitine is produced in the liver and kidneys from the essential amino acids lysine and methionine. Although not essential, it is very often deficient in vegetarians, whose diets contain low levels of lysine and methionine. Beef and pork, rich sources, are unhealthy for many other reasons. L-carnitine maximizes the amount of oxygen that the heart and skeletal muscle can extract from blood. Skeletal muscle has up to seventy times the l-carnitine of blood plasma. It prevents the accumulation of long-chain fatty acids in heart muscle by improving their oxidation and conversion into energy and it is the only nutrient that can do this.[63]

Low levels of l-carnitine are associated with impaired, inefficient heart function. It works in the inner mitochondrial membrane to reduce arrhythmia, lower the risk of heart failure, and relieve cramping in the lower extremities. Of tremendous importance is the fact that l-carnitine assists in the production of ATP, also produced in mitochondria, and preserves the on-hand supply. This is important since the heart gets 60 percent of its energy from fat source tissue. Deficiencies of l-carnitine have been observed in people with heart disease. L-carnitine is also a powerful antioxidant. It reduces and prevents the death of heart muscle and surrounding tissue while lowering the risk and occurrence of arrhythmias. L-carnitine is nontoxic and very well tolerated.

Our Recommended Daily Amount: 500 mg, three times daily.

L-Gluthathione

This is a uniquely powerful compound found in all living cells. L-gluthathione is considered the most potent member of the body's detoxification system and is an intensely aggressive antioxidant. One of the first antioxidants incorporated into plant life billions of years ago, it is a master free radical scavenger.

Synthesized from the amino acid cysteine, its primary role is an antioxidant against synthetic and natural oxidants. It prevents the oxidation (biological rusting) of fats, called lipid peroxidation. This peroxidation is extremely dangerous because it damages and destroys cell membranes, crucial in regard to the endothelial lining of the arteries leading from your heart. L-gluthathione, as part of the GSH (reduced gluthathione) peroxidase enzyme complex, reduces and destroys lipid peroxides, prevents unsaturated fats from oxidizing, and prevents cell membrane damage.[64] It is also a red blood cell protector.

Our Recommended Daily Amount: follow directions on Supplement Facts panel.

L-Lysine

An essential amino acid, lysine is found in all plant and animal foods. Levels of l-lysine are much higher in animal foods, which contain high levels of saturated fat. The cooking process oxidizes these saturated fats, making them more dangerous for the heart. This suggests that l-lysine should be taken supplementally. L-lysine is critical to the formation of hydroxylysine in Type III collagen found in arterial tissue, and will replace incomplete and structurally weak lysyl residues in the collagen of arterial connective tissues to help strengthen them and prevent arterial injury. It is also a precursor of l-carnitine and acetyl CoA, critical for carbohydrate metabolism.

Our Recommended Daily Amount: 1,000 mg, three times daily.

L-Proline and Hydroxyproline

L-proline is the third most concentrated free amino acid in the body fluids of adults. It is considered a nonessential amino acid, yet it plays a vital role in the production of healthy collagen and should be considered essential. Proline is found in collagen, which makes up about 25 to 30 percent of the body's proteins. It has been determined that about 50 percent of our proline is stored in collagen. Proline, like lysine, will replace incomplete and structurally weak collagen residues, helping to strengthen them and prevent arterial injury.

Our Recommended Daily Amount: 500 mg, two to three times daily.

Lycopene

Tomato power! Lots of recent research clearly points out that lycopene is one of the most potent and powerful antioxidant carotenoids found in plant foods, with a particular ability to quench the extremely dangerous singlet oxygen. Research data shows that lycopene is clinically proven as a highly effective antioxidant against LDL oxidation. It is found in high concentration in tomatoes and tomato products. Tomato extracts also contain naturally occurring vitamin E, beta-carotene, cholesterol-lowering phytosterols, and the lycopene precursors phytoene and phytofluene. Lycopene is one of the three most prevalent carotenoids in blood, yet we cannot produce it internally. Diets rich in lycopene have been shown to reduce the risk of certain cancers—prostate, mouth, pharynx, esophagus, stomach, and colon. Studies show it reduces the risk of cervical cancer fivefold.

Our Recommended Daily Amount: 50 to 100 mg, once daily.

Magnesium

This essential macromineral, second most abundant in the body, is naturally found in tofu, legumes, green leafy vegetables, whole grains, nuts, and seeds. Magnesium plays a vital role in hundreds of biochemical processes and metabolic pathways, is a required component of more than three hundred enzymes, and is critical for heart health.

Magnesium is vital to heart muscle contraction, muscle relaxation, and blood clotting, and is essential for the production of ATP. There is about ten times as much magnesium in heart muscle cells as there is in blood. Unfortunately, magnesium is lacking in our diet.

A 1971 article in the *American Journal of Clinical Nutrition* stated that when whole wheat is refined to make white flour, 85 percent of the magnesium is removed.[65] This makes it difficult to obtain the Daily Value of 400 milligrams, still an insufficient amount for cardiovascular health. Stress causes magnesium depletion by the action of adrenaline and cortisol causing it to be released from cells and excreted into urine. Type-A personalities produce more adrenaline and cortisol; consequently, more magnesium is lost.[66]

Certain types of heart medications, such as thiazide diuretics, loop diuretics, chemotherapy drugs, digoxin, and cortisone deplete magnesium. Low magnesium levels and magnesium deficiency caused by a lower than normal dietary intake can be a strong risk factor for hypertension, cardiac arrhythmias, ischemic heart disease, atherogenesis, and sudden cardiac death. A review study by B. Altura at the Department of Physiology, State University of New York, Health Science Center, Brooklyn, indicated that magnesium plays a controlling role in the balance of blood fats and fat uptake by macrophages and how they will attach to the vessel wall.[67] Magnesium alone can inhibit platelet clumping in the same way that aspirin does without the gastrointestinal side effects. It blocks calcium channels to prevent tightening of arteries, promotes dilation of blood vessels, and enhances fibrinolytic (clotting) activity. Plus, magnesium can improve the efficiency of heart muscle cell function, allowing heart muscle that is deprived of oxygen to function with less oxygen. This is critical during cardiac stress situations: maximizing cellular metabolism makes the difference between cells living and cells dying.

In 1960, Nobel Prize winner Hans Selye, M.D., demonstrated the ability of magnesium to protect the heart from damage. His famous study proved that rats fed a supposedly adequate level of magnesium all developed heart attacks. Of those fed additional magnesium, only twenty-nine had MIs (myochardial infarctions).[68] A 1985 study carried out at the Georgetown University College of Medicine illustrated that cardiac muscle is more susceptible to injury when there is a serum deficiency of magnesium resulting from insufficient dietary intake.

We can look at numerous studies conducted from 1958 through the late 1990s that show magnesium given during heart attacks can save lives.[69] Current therapy uses clot-busters like warfarin (Coumadin) combined with aspirin and heparin to thin the blood. But magnesium is safer and does not cause bleeding or side effects. It blocks calcium uptake and relaxes blood vessels in the same way that ACE (angiotensin-converting enzyme) inhibitors do.

Magnesium deficiency always accompanies diabetes. It is also directly correlated to the severity of angina.[70] As a natural calcium channel blocker, magnesium prevents the entry of excess calcium into heart cells, which can cause the heart to spasm. Magnesium is a potent antispasmodic mineral that relaxes blood vessels, prevents heart and arterial spasms, and enables blood to flow through the arteries with less resistance, resulting in lower pressure. Magnesium in the form of magnesium chloride is a primary emergency room treatment when someone is having a heart attack and can stop it.

Our Recommended Daily Amount: 400 to 800 mg for prevention; 800 to 1,200 mg for cardiovascular problems. Suggested forms are magnesium citrate or chelated magnesium.

MSM (Methylsulfonylmethane)

MSM is an organic form of the element sulfur that is naturally found in our bodies and nature. It is an integral component of the atmosphere, the soil, and the oceans. Scientists value it as an essential player in the sulfur cycle needed for life.

MSM comes from microscopic plankton that release sulfur into the seawater. This rapidly changes to a volatile gas called *dimethyl sulfide* (DMS), which then heads up into the atmosphere. Ultraviolet light rays and ozone change the DMS to dimethyl sulfoxide (DMSO) and then to DMSO-2, known as MSM. This drops to the ground and is absorbed by plants. After all this, only traces, just a few parts per million, make their way into edible foods, such as fruits, vegetables, and grains.

MSM is also heat sensitive and is destroyed in cooking. It is required in every living cell and vitally contributes to the functions of enzymes, antibodies, antioxidants, and hormones. Because MSM is essential to these biological processes, we must get a continuous supply.

The nutritional benefits of MSM were discovered and documented by Robert J. Herschler in the early 1980s. About the same time, Stanley W. Jacob, M.D., at the Oregon Health Sciences University, began studying the bionutritional actions of MSM. Its functions are numerous. Proteins in hair, skin, and nails (keratin and collagen) and the formation of ligaments, tendons, bones, and joints are some of the main functions of this essential structural compound. It is also needed to produce insulin in the pancreas.[71] MSM also contributes to gastrointestinal health and provides resistance to allergens.

According to Craig Weatherby and Leonid Gordin, M.D., authors of *The Arthritis Bible*, the main function and benefit of MSM for the heart and cardiovascular system is the ability to donate its sulfur atoms for the purpose of constructing Type III collagen. This is vital, along with vitamin C, lysine, and proline, to form strong arteries, blood vessels, and other connective tissue and enzymes.[72] Recent studies indicate that MSM has powerful anti-inflammatory properties that can be quite effective at reducing arterial inflammation. Some people confuse biological sulfur (MSM), which is a nutrient, with sulfa drugs (synthetic pharmaceutical drugs used as antibiotics) and sulfites used in the preparation of foods and in wine. If you are allergic to sulfa drugs or sulfites, you won't be allergic to MSM.

Our Recommended Daily Amount: 500 mg, three times daily of 99 percent pure MSM with 34 percent bioavailable sulfur. *Do not take with blood thinners like heparin.*

Niacin

This essential B vitamin, also known as B$_3$, has been shown for years to lower cholesterol. The use of niacin to lower cholesterol was initially discussed in the 1950s. In fact, over the years, niacin has proven to be a more effective cholesterol-lowering agent than cholesterol-lowering drugs. Many doctors still don't prescribe niacin before drugs although the evidence is strong. This was shown in a fifteen-year mortality study of the long-term benefits of niacin by P. L. Canner, reported in 1986 in the *Journal of the American College of Cardiology*.[73]

Even after the Coronary Drug Project examined the effectiveness of cholesterol-lowering drugs, niacin was singled out as the only one to reduce mortality from cardiovascular disease. As further strong evidence, the study published in the *Annals of Internal Medicine* in 1994 concluded over a twenty-six-week period that niacin was an effective cholesterol-lowering agent. It lowered LDL cholesterol 5 percent after ten weeks and 23 percent after twenty-six weeks. It also raised HDL cholesterol 20 percent after ten weeks and 33 percent after twenty-six weeks. Finally, and very significant, was its effect on lipoprotein(a): levels of lipoprotein(a) dropped 14 percent in ten weeks and 35 percent in twenty-six weeks.[74] Very effective! It also lowers LDL, triglycerides, and fibrinogen, and raises HDL.

Since there are several forms of niacin available, the correct one must be used. The safest and most effective form of niacin is inositol hexaniacinate—"no-flush" niacin. In this form, it safely lowers cholesterol without the discomforting flush caused by the other forms. The niacinamide form causes a flushing of the skin after about twenty minutes and therefore large quantities cannot be taken. The time-released form is reported to cause a toxic effect on the liver.

Our Recommended Daily Amount: 500 mg, three times daily.

Plant Sterols (Beta-Sitosterol, Campesterol, and Stigmasterol)

Sterols are fatlike substances found in food and made in the body. The best-known sterol is cholesterol, made by the liver. But plants appear to provide richer, healthier sources. Full-fat soy foods, polyunsaturated vegetable oils (particularly unrefined, nonhydrogenated soybean oil), and legumes are rich sources. The three main plant sterols found in foods are beta-sitosterol, campesterol, and stigmasterol.

Beta-sitosterol is the main phytosterol in oils and legumes. Plant sterols are exciting substances for heart health because they have been shown to lower cholesterol levels. A Canadian study done by P. J. Jones and colleagues demonstrated that phytosterols work by blocking the absorption of dietary cholesterol and preventing the production of cholesterol in the liver.[75] Because they are less well absorbed than animal source cholesterol, they have no side effects as do cholesterol-lowering drugs. And it appears that only small amounts of the phytosterols are necessary to lower cholesterol. Studies show that less than 1 gram per day will do the trick.[76] And just recently, the FDA authorized a claim for the effectiveness of plant sterols and stanols, stating that they may lower the risk of heart disease. According to the FDA, 1.3 grams of plant sterols or 3.4 grams of plant stanols in combination with a diet low in saturated fat and cholesterol lowers cholesterol.

Our Recommended Daily Amount: 100 mg, three times daily for preventive use, and 400 to 500 mg, three times daily, to lower cholesterol.

Potassium

This is a magical mineral for the cardiovascular system and blood. There is nothing else in nature that effectively lowers blood pressure as well as potassium. It is the natural sodium and high blood pressure antagonist. Many experts believe that high blood pressure is caused in great part by the ratio of potassium to sodium in the diet and, consequently, in the blood. A diet that is plant based is rich in potassium and low in sodium. Conversely, an animal-based diet that is rich in sodium is low in potassium. When the ratio of potassium to sodium is high, between 4:1 and 20:1, blood pressure will remain low. When the ratio of potassium to sodium is low or reversed, between 1:1 and 1:20, blood pressure will be high. With today's high consumption of meats and processed foods loaded with sodium and much less consumption of plant foods, fruits, vegetables, grains, and legumes, it's no wonder ratios are out of whack.

Our Recommended Daily Amount: 3,000 to 5,000 mg from dietary sources.

Quercetin

This active bioflavonoid found in red onions and grapefruit increases the duration of effectiveness and the activity level of vitamin C. Quercetin has a strong stabilizing effect on cell membranes and actively counters the destructive action in diabetic retinopathy and promotes the secretion of insulin, and is a potent inhibitor of sorbitol accumulation, particularly in the eyes of diabetics. Reducing sorbitol prevents diabetic retinopathy and macular degeneration.

Our Recommended Daily Amount: 50 to 100 mg daily.

Red Yeast Rice (*Monascus purpureaus*)

This funny-sounding supplement is actually a food staple in many Asian countries that has been consumed for quite some time. Red yeast rice inhibits the metabolic activity of the enzyme 3-hydroxy 3-methylglutaryl-coenzyme A (HMG-CoA reductase) that is responsible for producing cholesterol in the liver.

Red koji, a type of red yeast grown on fermented rice and oatmeal in Japan, contains a natural statin compound called monacolin K (lovastatin). Red koji is biochemically similar to pharmaceutical cholesterol-lowering statins, such as Zocor and Mevacor, that block HMG-CoA reductase but without the side effects. This blocking action effectively reduces total cholesterol and LDL cholesterol levels in the blood. In one study, cholesterol levels decreased 18 to 35 percent without changing HDL levels.

Our Recommended Daily Amount: 1200 mg, two times daily. *Not recommended with liver disease, serious infection, or after surgery.*

Resveratrol

The French people consume large quantities of fatty foods high in saturated fats and cholesterol. Yet their mortality rate from coronary heart disease is much lower than in other cultures. They have only one-third the mortality rate compared to the average of other cultures. Based on this phenomenon, referred to as the French paradox, a resurgence of interest recently focused on the roles of wine, bioflavonoids, proanthocyanidins, and resveratrol in the prevention of cardiovascular disease.

The main causes of death from coronary heart disease are heart attack, increased blood-clotting activity, and atherosclerosis. Atherosclerosis causes cerebrovascular and cardiovascular disease that leads to ischemic strokes and heart attacks, thereby responsible for more than 40 percent of all deaths in Western civilization.[77,78]

Resveratrol has many cardioprotective benefits. The pioneering research of C. Pace-Asciak has led us to understand that resveratrol, a polyphenol found in wine and other foods, has a powerful ability to block the clumping of platelets in the blood.[79] It also reduced thromboxane A_2 production in human blood platelet cells by approximately 60 percent. Thromboxane A_2 is a powerful eicosanoid produced from arachidonic acid (an omega-6 derivative) that is involved in the development of blood platelet aggregation. Neither quercitin nor any of the other phytochemicals or antioxidants in wine had any effect at this concentration.[80] And wine-source resveratrol inhibited platelet aggregation of healthy human blood plasma, although the antiplatelet activity of ethanol (grain alcohol) has been incorrectly advanced as one of the mechanisms involved in wine's protection against cardiovascular disease.[81] Platelet aggregation of healthy human blood plasma decreased by more than 50 percent with resveratrol. Red wine containing natural trans-resveratrol and polyphenols inhibited platelet aggregation by 41.9 percent. By increasing resveratrol concentrations in wine, inhibition of platelet aggregation was raised to 78.5 percent.

Resveratrol reduces serum cholesterol and triglyceride levels. Studies confirm that it inhibited deposition of cholesterol and triglycerides in the liver, reduced levels of serum triglycerides and low-density lipoprotein (LDL) cholesterol, and reduced the total cholesterol/high-density lipoprotein (HDL) cholesterol ratio.[82]

Moreover, resveratrol initiates both direct and indirect blood pressure–lowering effects on arteries by stimulating nitric oxide production and other mechanisms that dilate them. At one concentration, vasorelaxation by resveratrol was reversible. At a higher concentration, vasorelaxation by resveratrol could not be reversed, demonstrating that resveratrol acts directly to relax vascular smooth muscle cells.[83]

It also has antioxidant effects and protects against free radical injury *In Vivo* (in the body). The 1997 *Neuroreport* study supported the hypothesis that resveratrol reduced oxidative stress and increased the antioxidant protective effects of vitamins C and E.[84] It also protects against free radical injury in cerebral ischemia (mini-strokes). Administration of polydatin, a plant-derived form of resveratrol, decreased levels of certain free radicals and increased the antioxidant activity of superoxide dismutase (SOD), catalase, and gluthathione peroxidase.[85] It increased plasma HDL and enhanced antioxidant activity as judged by decreased levels of LDL lipid peroxides and total peroxides.[86] Resveratrol is a potent inhibitor of LDL cholesterol, lowering the oxidation rate by 81 percent. In contrast, alpha-tocopherol (natural vitamin E), which has been associated with a reduced risk of heart disease, had a much lower antioxidant potency than resveratrol, inhibiting LDL cholesterol oxidation by only 40 percent.[87]

Another form of resveratrol is a trans-resveratrol extract produced from the traditional Chinese medicinal herb *Polygonum cuspidatum*. It is even more potent, containing one thousand times more resveratrol than wine or grape-derived ingredients. Spectacular!

Our Recommended Daily Amount: follow directions on Supplement Facts panel.

Selenium

This micromineral is essential for the prevention of disease and the maintenance of optimal health. It is very important to supplement the diet with selenium because it is found in low quantities or is nonexistent in many soils throughout the country. A low level of selenium has been positively associated in the research studies with an increased risk of cardiovascular disease. Selenium is a powerful detoxifying antioxidant that works in the gluthathione detoxification mechanism of the liver.[88] It has powerful scavenging abilities that protect arterial cells from being attacked by free radicals. A 1989 study conducted by Frans Kok in the Department of Epidemiology at Erasmus University Medical School, Rotterdam, the Netherlands, found that patients in a study group who suffered from heart attacks had a dramatically lower level of selenium than patients in a control group that did not have a history of heart attack.[89]

Our Recommended Daily Amount: 200 mcg in the l-selenomethionine form.

Soy Isoflavones

Soy is a fully loaded mixed bag of heart-healthy phytonutrients and a rich nutritional feast for the body. Recently, soy owes its much of its skyrocketing consumption to the fact that it has been shown as health promoting for a variety of health concerns. In October 1999, a health claim made for soy was accepted and approved by the FDA. This claim can now be become part of a dietary supplement or functional food's label.

Abundant in uniquely beneficial bioflavonoids called isoflavones (genistein, daidzein, and glycitein), soy has demonstrated success as a heart-healthy supplement or addition to the diet. The isoflavones in soy are powerful antioxidants. Q. H. Meng conducted a study supporting this claim in 1999. It confirmed that isoflavones in soy increased the resistance of LDL cholesterol to oxidation.[90] Many researchers believe that 30 to 60 mg of isoflavones per day can reduce cholesterol. John R. Rouse III and colleagues at the Wake Forest University School of Medicine in Winston Salem, North Carolina, conducted another interesting study. It confirmed that soy isoflavones do lower LDL cholesterol and total cholesterol, although the mechanism by which soy accomplishes this is not yet understood; it is believed to be the action of the protein itself. Using different diets, some with casein as the protein, only the diet with soy protein and soy isoflavones combined was able to reduce cholesterol.[91]

Soy isoflavones can ease menopausal symptoms (especially hot flashes) because they are also phytoestrogens (mild plant versions of human estrogens). The omega-3 and omega-6 EFAs also take credit for turning soy into a powerful natural cholesterol-lowering and heart-healthy extra in the diet. That's not all. Soy is a rich source of lecithin, a well-known natural fat emulsifier containing phosphatidylcholine, capable of breaking down cholesterol, triglycerides, and other fats in the blood. Soy is also rich in healthy plant protein (about one-third of the bean) and provides all eight essential amino acids plus many others.

What about GMOs (genetically modified organisms)? As we discussed earlier, soy is the rage, but can we count on it to be GMO free? Not yet, say the experts. Although a growing number of soy supplements and food products are already GMO free, we can't clearly know without testing whether or not they're tainted. How to know for sure? Manufacturers are beginning to buy their beans from certified GMO–free crops. They are testing them at independent third-party–certification labs. They can then clearly and confidently label their products as third-party–certified GMO free. As for organic soybeans, it is also incorrect to assume that they are definitely GMO–free simply because they are organic. While it's less likely that organic soy products contain GMOs because organic producers are considerably more concerned about "unnatural" substances in or on the beans and their growing environment, this is still no guarantee. Nature's simple process of cross-pollination can transfer GMOs from one crop to another quite easily.

Our Recommended Daily Amount: Soy isoflavones, 50 to 100 mg.

Soy Lecithin and Soy Phospholipids

Lecithin, the old "fat buster" favorite, has been around since the beginning of dietary supplement days. It has legendary fat- and cholesterol-emulsifying properties. It contains the phospholipids PC (phosphatidylcholine) and PS (phophatidylserine).

Phospholipids are major components of all cell membranes. Soy phosphatidylserine is a phospholipid found in soy that improves memory, lifts depression, and lessens Alzheimer's symptoms by promoting and preserving cell membrane fluidity and integrity in the brain. It is often found combined with other memory enhancers like ginkgo biloba. Soy phosphatidylcholine is another soy phospholipid that increases the solubility of cholesterol while promoting and maintaining cellular health.

Our Recommended Daily Amount: follow directions on Supplement Facts panel.

Spirulina

Spirulina is one of approximately fifteen hundred species of microscopic aquatic plants called blue-green microalgae that have inhabited the earth for several million years. Anthropologists and biologists believe that spirulina is the oldest plant on earth. This "old faithful" source of health from the sea has provided complete nutrition, unmatched in value, for over three and one-half million years. Only in the past seventy-five years have we become familiar with spirulina, a powder keg of green power that has the potential, along with other blue-green and green algae, to become the prime choice for a world superfood of the future.

There are two common varieties of this spiral-shaped blue-green algae currently being cultivated and harvested for human consumption, known as spirulina maxima and spirulina platensis. In its natural state, spirulina is primarily found in the salt-rich lakes, seas, and waterways of Africa, Central America, and South America. Hundreds of years ago, the Aztecs of Mexico regularly harvested spirulina for food from natural green lakes and ponds. Native cooks mixed it with maize (cornmeal) to make green pancakes that were a staple of their simple diet. Spirulina is also grown and cultivated in tank environments that are set up to provide growing conditions that mimic its ideal natural habitat.

Hawaiian spirulina is harvested in tanks and in natural saltwater seashore coves, where the mineral composition of the salt water is ideally suited for growing and many hours of intense sunlight each day produce rapid growth. Immediately after being scooped out of the water, it is filtered to a thick consistency and flash-frozen to preserve its nutrients. It is then dried, ground into a powder, and processed.

Perhaps the largest spirulina "farm" is located in the California desert, far away from polluted city air. This controlled environment keeps out undesirable weed algae, microbacteria, and parasites. When removed from the tanks, it is dehydrated and readied for use in dietary supplements.

Spirulina has been blessed by nature with a huge arsenal of valuable nutrients. Of special interest is phycocyanin, which is present in large amounts. Results of a 1986 study presented at the International Association for Dental Research General Session concluded that phycocyanin was unique because of its cytostatic (suppressing formation of new cancer cell colonies) and cytotoxic (destroying existing colonies of cancer cells) abilities. Spirulina is naturally "pumped" with vitamins, especially the carotenoids like beta-carotene. It contains minerals, EFAs, the important fatty acid gamma linolenic acid (GLA), and natural digestive enzymes. And it's a complete protein, with all eight essential amino acids present. Spirulina is about four times as rich in protein (60 percent) as beef (18 percent). In our society, where the concept of complete protein is meat and dairy, it is very reassuring to know that greens such as spirulina can provide high-quality protein and other nutrients.

Spirulina's cell wall is unique, too. It is made up of mucopolysaccharides that provide numerous health benefits. Among them is the ability to lower blood fats. At the Avinashilingam Institute for Home Science, Deemed University in Coimbatore, India, A. Ramamoorthy and colleagues tested the effects of spirulina on patients with a combination of high cholesterol (above 250 mg/dl) and ischemic heart disease. They concluded that spirulina plays a key role, lowering blood cholesterol levels and improving lipid profiles.[92] This was also brought to light in a 1976 study showing that spirulina controlled the tendency and ability of cholesterol and other lipoproteins to bond with arterial receptors and attach to artery walls.

As a food additive, spirulina maxima contains beta-carotene, tocopherols, and phenolic acids, which are proven to exhibit antioxidant properties. The M. S. Miranda study, recently published in the

216

Brazilian *Journal of Medical and Biological Research*, demonstrated a 71 percent antioxidant capacity for the group taking the spirulina extract and 54 percent for the group that did not, indicating strong antioxidant protection.[93] The antioxidant activity of spirulina can be attributed to phycocyanin, the blue pigment found in blue-green algae that contains phytochemicals with scavenging properties. The C. Romay study demonstrated that phycocyanin is able to scavenge the very dangerous hydroxy radical and inhibit the oxidation of lipids in the liver.[94]

Spirulina also lowers blood pressure. Research studies show that spirulina was able to cause a significant change in vascular tone by increasing the synthesis and release of nitric oxide and by decreasing the synthesis and release of a vasoconstricting substance from the endothelial cells.[95]

A major argument frequently used to support the consumption of animal foods in the diet incorrectly states that plants do not contain vitamin B_{12}. Spirulina does contain some. That's good news and reassuring for vegetarians who incorrectly believe that eating animal food is critical to getting this essential blood-building vitamin.

Our Recommended Daily Amount: Although no guidelines have been established at this time, many experts suggest about 10,000 mg per day as a preventive dose. For therapeutic use, up to 20,000 mg per day is indicated.

TMG (Trimethylglycine, or Betaine)

TMG (betaine—not to be confused with betaine hydrochloride, the digestive acid) is a phytonutrient found in many plants and marine invertebrates. Beets are the richest source. TMG is the best-known source of methyl groups and is the best methyl donor. You will recall that methylation is a process whereby methyl groups attach to our DNA and prevent the formation of defective genes, those that produce disease or disorders, from occurring. TMG plays a significant role in promoting heart health, preventing aging, and more. Methyl groups also convert the cardioirritant homocysteine to harmless methionine, reducing homocysteine levels in the blood. Although TMG is not considered essential, it should be because although we can produce it from choline, we do not produce sufficient amounts for optimum cardiovascular health. A diet rich in beets, broccoli, and spinach can provide over 500 mg per day. TMG is also a lipotropic substance that improves fat metabolism, decreases levels of dangerous VLDLs, and builds muscle mass while reducing body fat.

Our Recommended Daily Amount: 500 mg.

Vanadium

Vanadium, a micromineral, is not essential, but many experts consider it to be. It appears to mimic the activity of insulin. This biochemical behavior seems to improve glucose management in insulin-dependent diabetics. Type II diabetics benefit from its ability to improve glucose tolerance and lower glucose levels.[96] And a report by B. F. Arland in the *Journal of the American Dietetic Association* states that vanadium seems to inhibit the production of cholesterol.[97]

According to a 1993 study in the *Industrial Journal of Biochemistry*, Nandhini was convinced that the BGOV (bis-glycinato-oxo-vanadium), an organic form of vanadium, offered superior efficacy and bioavailability.

Our Recommended Daily Amount: follow directions on Supplement Facts panel.

Vitamin C

Here's a supplement that requires a whole book to discuss. In fact, several whole books, such as *Vitamin C: The Master Nutrient* by Sandra Goodman, Ph.D., and *Cancer and Vitamin C* by Linus Pauling, Ph.D., and Ewan Cameron, M.D., have been written about vitamin C. There are literally thousands of scientific studies and research papers that unquestionably support the cardiovascular and general health-promoting roles and functions of vitamin C.

Found in citrus fruits, tomatoes, peppers, broccoli, and other vegetables, it is the primary water-soluble antioxidant in the body. Because we cannot produce vitamin C internally, we must obtain it from food and supplemental sources. Thousands of studies clearly support vitamin C's ability to protect against free radical damage. As an antioxidant, vitamin C attacks, neutralizes, and destroys reactive oxygen species. It scavenges superoxide and hydroxyl radicals.[98] Studies show than vitamin C works with vitamin E to prevent the free radical chain oxidation of lipids.[99] Vitamin C also regenerates vitamin E. It increases rate at which cholesterol is removed by conversion to bile acids. Vitamin C inhibits oxidation of LDL cholesterol and increases the HDL cholesterol and triglyceride levels.

Vitamin C was known to be essential for collagen synthesis more than fifty years ago. Incredibly, the Bartlett study in 1942 explained that vitamin C deficiency is responsible for weakening blood vessels and heart.[100] Its role has been intensely studied by Dr. Anthony Verlangieri, Director of the Atherosclerosis Research Laboratories at the University of Mississippi. He believes vitamin C is essential with vitamin E to make GAGs (glucosaminoglycans), the crucial ingredient of the "glue" that holds arterial cells in place.[101] Verlangieri explains that deficiencies of vitamin C cause deterioration of cell linings that result in arterial injuries that attract cholesterol and initiate atherosclerosis.[102] In another study, Verlangieri determined that arteries with high vitamin C levels have lower cholesterol levels and a reversal of atherosclerosis.[103] In 1944, Rogoff disclosed, in the *Pennsylvania Medical Journal*, the ability of vitamin C to potentiate the activity of insulin.[104] Vitamin C also forms a synergistic defense partnership by both regenerating and increasing the effectiveness of vitamin E.[105]

Vitamin C reduces stress. A study presented at the August 1999 meeting of the American Chemical Society in New Orleans by M. O'Keefe and colleagues related that rats induced with stress and then given 200 mg of vitamin C daily had lower levels of glucocorticoids (stress hormones) compared with those who did not receive the C. This simply affirmed that vitamin C prevents stress.[106]

Vitamin C is nature's best cardiovascular protection. It is considered essential for dozens of metabolic functions. While all are truly vital, the most essential one is the formation of your body's primary and predominant connective tissue protein—collagen. By taking a major role in the formation of collagen, vitamin C builds a strong yet flexible collagen matrix in our arteries, making them resistant to pressure and the attacks of free radicals and other irritating substances. It lowers serum cholesterol. Vitamin C also increases the activity and effectiveness of the immune system, thereby reducing stress and the excess adrenalin that stress produces.

Take "C" and see. Truly the body's master water-soluble nutrient, vitamin C is the most effective free radical–scavenging antioxidant for the eyes. In the eye its most important function is to manufacture collagen to strengthen connective tissue. Collagen promotes the development of healthy retinal capillaries that deliver antioxidants and other nutrients to prevent free radical damage in the lens. In clinical studies, vitamin C has also demonstrated the ability to reduce intraocular pressure, which is common in glaucoma.

Despite thousands of positive studies, there is always some controversy about the value of vitamin C. A 1999 article in *Better Nutrition* by Associate Editor, Patty Andersen Parrado examined one of the latest attacks against vitamin C. Her article, "Vitamin C: Friend or Foe?" discussed recent news presented at the American Heart Association's fortieth Annual Conference on Cardiovascular Disease, Epidemiology, and Prevention. The premise that vitamin C supplementation may increase one's risk of developing atherosclerosis certainly came as a surprise.

Interestingly, this paper had not yet been published in a peer-reviewed medical journal and there were prominent nutrition experts who cast doubt on the findings. The essence of it was this: Researchers measured the thickness of an arterial wall in the necks of 573 healthy men aged forty to sixty over an eighteen-month period. Men who took 500 mg of vitamin C daily had an increase in arterial wall thickness that was two and one-half times greater than men who did not use supplements. Yet this unpublished study was in direct conflict with a 1995 study in the American Heart Association journal, *Circulation*. That research found a significant reduction in carotid artery wall thickness in people over age fifty-five who consumed about 1,000 mg or more of vitamin C a day, compared to those consuming less than 88 mg per day.

Parrado went on to tell readers about a press release issued by Oregon State University vitamin C expert, Balz Frei, professor and director of the university's Linus Pauling Institute. He explained, "The results from the study, in fact, are in direct conflict with a study published in 1995 and the findings of the *Circulation* study were based on more than eleven thousand people and, unlike the more recent study, had undergone rigorous peer review before publication." Frei added that over twenty clinical studies since 1996 have consistently observed beneficial effects of vitamin C, advising that "the known health benefits of vitamin C far outweigh alleged, unconfirmed risks."

Although most of the research focuses on vitamin C as an antioxidant, it is also a pro-oxidant as demonstrated by its ability to be toxic to bacteria, viruses, and certain cells, such as malignant cancer cells (but it is far less toxic to normal cells).

Our Recommended Daily Amount: 500 to 1,000 mg, three times daily. Do not take all your vitamin C at one time. It is water soluble and the body will excrete the unused portion.

Vitamin E

Vitamin E, the premier fat-soluble vitamin in the body, is naturally found in green leafy vegetables, soy, legumes, nuts, seeds, unrefined vegetable oils, and whole grains. It was discovered during the 1920s while conducting fertility experiments in rats.

Many of us think that vitamin E is just one substance, while it is actually eight. There are four tocopherols and four tocotrienols. Interestingly, the word *tocopherol* is derived from the Greek "to give birth." Of the four tocopherols, named alpha, beta, gamma, and delta, the alpha, or d-alpha form, is most common.

Thousands of studies have been conducted on vitamin E and its functions, activities, and roles in human nutrition and health. The message is clear. In its natural d-alpha tocopherol form it is a potent, aggressive free radical–scavenging antioxidant, the activity of which prevents cellular damage by destroying free radicals before they have a chance to destroy cell membranes. Vitamin E is also a powerful blood thinner, accomplishing this by preventing the clumping (aggregation) of platelets in the blood. It increases circulation, drops blood pressure, and accelerates the healing of scar tissue. It also acts as an antioxidant in fat-containing tissues, specifically cell membranes.

Vitamin E directly protects against heart disease by guarding lipoproteins, the carriers of cholesterol. It prevents lipid peroxidation (the biological rusting of fats), specifically the oxidation of LDL cholesterol, which easily sticks to artery walls. Vitamin E also halts the progression of free radical chain reactions, by preventing free radical damage. A study by Gerald Reaven in 1993 explained that people taking 1,600 mg per day of vitamin E achieved a 50 percent reduction of LDL cholesterol.[107]

Vitamin E also prevents abnormal thickening of the blood, which can cause clotting, by forming a slippery coating on the artery lining to maintain a smooth flow of blood.[108] Red blood cell health is also promoted with vitamin E. The current Daily Value for vitamin E is only 30 IU, far too little to reap the benefits of its optimum cardiovascular protective effects and overall protective abilities. A study using over 87,000 nurses found that those who received 100 IU of vitamin E daily for two years reduced their risk of heart disease by 41 percent.[109] And a 39,000-person study of male health care professionals turned up a similar finding—more than 30 IU of vitamin E each day produced a 37 percent lower risk of CVD than that of a control group who did not supplement.[110]

Vitamin E also prevents polyunsaturated fats from becoming oxidized. That's the verdict of Allison McEwan Jenkinson and her colleagues. Her study, published in the *FASEB Journal*, tells us that polyunsaturated fatty acids (PUFAs), such as those found in flax, corn, safflower oil, and fish, are extremely susceptible to oxidation by free radicals and need to be sufficiently protected in the diet. The study determined that levels of supplemental vitamin E, given at 120 IU daily, protected lymphocytes in the immune system against DNA damage caused by oxidation of PUFA in a PUFA–rich diet.[111] To effectively contribute to cardiovascular health, at least 400 to 1,000 IU are needed per day. Unfortunately, we cannot get anywhere near that much from out diets. Even diets rich in unprocessed vegetable oils, nuts, seeds, whole grains, and green leafy vegetables won't provide 100 IU.

At the Division of Hematology, Brown University, Memorial Hospital of Rhode Island, Manfred Steiner, M.D., Ph.D., studied the effect of vitamin E on platelet aggregation. At 400 IU per day, platelet aggregation was strongly inhibited by vitamin E, and at 1,200 IU per day, significantly prevented. This proved that vitamin E could be an effective inhibitor of platelet aggregation.[112]

In the Cambridge Heart Antioxidant Study, British researchers examined two thousand patients with angiographically proven coronary artery disease. One group received 400 to 800 IU of vitamin E per day or placebo for about eighteen months. The risk of having nonfatal heart attacks was decreased by 77 percent in those receiving the vitamin E. This clearly indicated that vitamin E can help prevent heart attacks in people who have been diagnosed with coronary artery disease.[113] Because vitamin E prevents blood from clotting, it reduces deposits from forming.[114]

Our Recommended Daily Amount: under age forty, 400 IU; over age forty, 400 to 800 IU. Take natural d-alpha tocopherol, preferably with mixed tocopherols, because synthetics have not been shown to exert the same potent antioxidant and blood thinning activity. Do not take more than 200 IU in combination with blood-thinning treatments, such as Coumadin, aspirin, EFAs, and gingko. Also advise your physician if you are currently on a blood thinner prior to combining its use with vitamin E.

Zinc

This essential mineral, found in whole grains, legumes, nuts, and seeds, is an integral part of more than two hundred enzyme reactions within the body and crucial to all aspects of blood sugar regulation. The production, secretion, and utilization of insulin are dependent upon zinc. Beta cells of the pancreas are protected by zinc. Because diabetics excrete large amounts of zinc in their urine, supplementation is essential and appears to benefit both Type I and Type II diabetics.[115]

Our Recommended Daily Amount: 15 mg for prevention and 15 to 30 mg for diabetics. Zinc supplementation is most effective in the forms of zinc L-monomethionine (chelated amino acid–bound zinc) and zinc citrate.

Systemic Oral Enzyme Therapy

It is clear from our earlier discussions that inflammation is a cause of and a warning sign for cardiovascular disease. As a cause, it evokes the immune response to produce white blood cells to fight inflammation and soak up cholesterol. As a warning sign, it tells us that arterial injury has occurred and has elevated C-reactive protein (CRP) in the blood. Inflammation triggers the body's response to repair and heal itself. This inflammation is easily reduced with systemic oral enzymes that help regenerate cells and improve the function of organs and tissues throughout the body. These enzymes are normally produced and used to break down food and deliver nutrients. When taken between meals, they reduce systemic inflammation. Oral enzymes should be taken regularly while monitoring blood levels of CRP. The most important and widely used systemic oral enzymes are:

- **Pancreatin**—a group of enzymes produced in the pancreas
- **Trypsin**—produced in the pancreas and boosts the immune system, accelerating the healing of injuries, and reducing the stickiness of blood
- **Chymotrypsin**—derived from animal sources, reduces blood stickiness
- **Bromelain**—derived from the pineapple core, inhibits platelet aggregation, strengthens the immune system, and has anti-inflammatory properties that activate metabolic activity, breaking down fibrin in inflamed tissue
- **Papain**—derived from papaya, has anti-inflammatory properties

Systemic oral enzyme therapy can destroy the main types of pathogens found in the blood that are related to heart disease, such as cytomegalovirus and *chlamydia pneumoniae*. Dr. Joseph Melnick of Baylor College of Medicine in Houston, Texas, has studied these bacterial renegades for seventeen years. Lesions from diseased arteries are typically found to contain cytomegalovirus, a common herpes virus. *Chlamydia pnuemoniae* has been implicated in triggering inflammation in tissues lining blood vessels that causes plaques. *Porphyromonas*, responsible for causing gum disease, also damages artery linings.

Dr. Raoul Garcia of the Boston Veterans Affairs Outpatient Clinic has examined more than 1,100 men over twenty-five years. All healthy at the start, those whose gums were the worst had twice the heart attack rate and three times the stroke rate of those with healthy gums. *Porphyromonas* has also been found in the carotid arteries. Wobenzyme N, the best-known and most studied systemic oral enzyme product, destroys bacteria that cause heart disease by stimulating the immune system to increase the formation of tumor necrosis factor (TNF), interleukin 1-b, and interleukin 6, which attack bacteria and viruses. Systemic oral enzymes increased the activity of macrophages by 700 percent and NK (natural killer cells) by 1,300 percent.[116] Systemic oral enzymes reduce inflammation and CRP levels after dental work.

At the Ukraine Scientific Institute of Cardiology, Kiev, Dr. I. K. Sledsewskaja noticed a significant drop in total cholesterol and LDL, decreased triglyceride formation, and a reduction in atherogenesis with the use of systemic oral enyzmes.[117] Wobenzyme N corrects immune status after a heart attack and reduces blood lipids.

Our Recommended Daily Amount: take between meals. Follow directions on Supplement Facts panel.

THIRTEEN

Exercise for Life

REGULAR EXERCISE BUILDS A HEALTHY HEART. ALONG WITH THE simple supplement and diet guidelines put forth so far, set your sights on a sensible plan to strengthen your heart with a combination of moderate, regular, long-term aerobic and anaerobic exercise. It increases levels of the antifat storage hormone glucagon, which reduces glucose and insulin levels and brings stored fats back into the blood to be metabolized for energy. At the same time, exercise reduces overall body fat and increases lean muscle mass, which is most efficient at burning fat. Keep in mind, however, that overexercising and overexertion can be dangerous.

Take a Hike for Health!

You've all heard it before and most of you don't like it! Exercise is repetitive body movement that improves the fitness, agility, tone, and fluidity of the body. However, exercise is essential to achieving, maintaining, and restoring optimal cardiovascular wellness and health. Your heart is your most important muscle. Exercise it often!

Exercise:

- Strengthens the heart and cardiovascular system by growing heart muscle and capillaries, thereby pumping more blood into the system with each beat while using less energy.
- Speeds up the metabolic rate by increasing the rate at which cells burn glucose and fat calories for energy.
- Increases the capacity of the lungs by increasing the amount of oxygen you take in and send into the bloodstrcam with each breath, ultimately requiring fewer breaths per minute and more efficient use of oxygen.
- Stimulates the immune system by activating the lymphatic system.
- Strengthens and increases the flexibility of muscles, bones, and connective and skin tissue.
- Improves sleep and defeats stress and depression by producing endorphins like serotonin that are natural pain-killing and sleep-inducing substances. It also creates a more physically exhausted state, which promotes better sleep and distracts attention from unpleasant thoughts.
- Metabolizes excess adrenaline, a very potent free radical oxidant substance.
- Reduces the need for insulin in the bloodstream.
- Improves digestion.
- Increases your energy level by using stored energy more efficiently.
- Accelerates weight loss.

Overexercising Is Bad for Your Health

However, you must be wise to the dangers of too much exercise, which can do the following:

- overwork the heart beyond its natural capacity,
- produce excess free radicals and consequently free radical damage,
- produce muscle strains and pains,
- cause dehydration in the absence of sufficient fluids to replace those lost through perspiration and exhaled breath,
- produce ketones, chemical substances that deplete iron. Ketogenic diets generate large amounts of uric acid from excessive protein metabolism. Ketones cause excess calcium excretion and fatigue.

Exercising for Weight Loss

To lose weight, you must burn adipose tissue (body fat), in order to reduce its overall percentage in the body. The amount of fat you burn depends upon the percentage of the maximum heart rate you achieve and sustain during your exercise session. Many people believe that exercising as hard and as fast as possible gives maximum weight-loss results—wrong!

First, the exercise must be aerobic (exercise that requires the cells to consume oxygen to produce energy). Aerobic exercise performed at 55 to 70 percent of your maximum heart rate burns the greatest amount of fat most efficiently, while giving the heart and cardiovascular system an excellent

What Is My Maximum Heart Rate?
220 − your age = your maximum heart rate (in beats per minute)

What Is My Target Heart Rate?
Your target heart rate = your maximum heart rate × the selected percentage (for your exercise goal)
Example: Age 46 for fat-burning workout
220 − 46 = 174 (maximum heart rate)
174 × 60 (60 percent selected percentage example for fat burning) = 104.4 (your target heart rate)

workout. The longer the duration of the workout, the greater its fat-burning ability becomes.

Exercise performed at more than 70 percent of your maximum heart rate burns more blood glucose and muscle/liver glycogen than fat. At this higher rate, the cardiovascular system achieves a superior workout compared to a fat-burning workout at the lower rate range.

Exercise Recommendations and Instructions

If you have a medical condition or are pregnant, check with your physician before beginning any exercise program.

We know that exercise is a "dirty word" to most of you who are usually too tired or busy to fit it in your schedule. However, obtaining cardiovascular health benefits is impossible without it. Quality aerobic exercise must be performed regularly. It is very important to choose a form of exercise that you can do consistently throughout the year, and requires little or no preparation and no special equipment or expense. Although walking, biking, jogging, swimming, dancing, rowing, and aerobics are good choices, we recommend walking. Why? The human species is bipedal—meaning that most movement is accomplished by walking on two feet. Therefore, walking on your two feet is the most natural form of exercise. Should you not choose walking as your primary form of exercise, choose one you enjoy, so you will look forward to doing it.

Walking Guidelines Begin your walk with stretching exercises or begin at an extremely slow pace for several minutes, to warm muscles and prevent injury. Gradually increase to the fastest comfortable pace you can maintain for the duration of your walk (follow your specific recommendations—see next section).

Measure your "perceived level of exertion" several times during your walk. To do this, become aware of how comfortable or uncomfortable you are during your walk on a scale of 1 to 10.

Perceived Level of Exertion

1–4   Low (little or no exertion)

5–7   Moderate (noticeable but not uncomfortable exertion)

8–10 High (heavy exertion, difficult breathing, pounding chest)

You can also measure your level of exertion by attempting conversation. If you experience difficulty speaking while you walk you are probably overexerting yourself and need to slow down. Toward the end of your walk, start slowing down your pace. For the last few minutes, walk slowly and do some stretching exercises upon completion to avoid muscle strain and injury. For walks of thirty minutes or longer, particularly in warm weather, make certain that you take along some water and drink 4 to 8 ounces every fifteen minutes to replenish lost fluids. Once again, be wise to the dangers of too much exercise.

Recommended Daily Walking Times

If you are 0 to 25 pounds over your target weight, walk:

15 minutes daily for the first week

30 minutes daily for the second week

45 minutes or more daily, for the rest of your life!

If you are 26 to 50 pounds over your target weight, walk:

10 minutes daily for the first week

20 minutes daily for the second week

30 minutes daily for the third week

45 minutes or more daily, for the rest of you life!

If you are 51+ pounds over your target weight, walk:

5 minutes daily for the first week

10 minutes daily for the second week

20 minutes daily for the third week

30 minutes daily for the fourth week

45 minutes or more daily, for the rest of your life!

If your current weight falls into this category and you feel the progression is too strenuous, continue at each stage for two weeks.

Plan on walking daily! Never allow more than one day off at a time, but don't walk if you are injured or ill.

FOURTEEN

De-Stress or Distress?

Learn to "Chill"

Stress kills! Excess adrenalin and cortisol production, induced by stress, along with the rise in blood pressure and heart rate it produces, damages the heart and cardiovascular system. And there's no such thing as a healthy heart without regular stress management. Understand that life naturally has its stressful situations, both positive and negative. These might include the death of a spouse, family member, or friend; marriage or divorce; the birth of a child; the loss of a job or a new job; retirement; sexual difficulties; a negative change in financial status; the onset of a serious health problem; and moving to a new residence.

Some degree of stress is not unhealthy. It is our response to the stresses we experience in life that may require improved coping techniques. Rest, relaxation, sufficient sleep, and a positive attitude are keys to de-stressing effectively. Learn to manage your stress so it does not become your distress.

Stress is a force or pressure that distorts the body, the thinking process, and emotions, and creates physical or mental tension, imbalance, and discomfort. The sources of stress can be either external or internal. Stress can be momentary, short term, or long term.

There are three types of stress:

- **Physical**: resulting from overwork, overexercising, injury, or lack of sleep.
- **Digestive**: resulting from eating unhealthy foods, overeating, or eating toxic foods and foods to which we are allergic.
- **Emotional**: resulting from personal, family, work, financial, or other problems and difficulties.

Volumes have been written about this subject. Many people wonder if it's true that stress kills and how it does so. Research tells us that the stress "fight or flight" response causes immediate biological changes within the body. The adrenal glands instantly begin producing adrenaline, glucagon, and cortisol. These hormones instruct the body to burn glucose at a faster rate for increased muscle energy. The rate of respiration increases, in order to take in more oxygen to burn the glucose. The heart pumps faster and harder to transport glucose and oxygen to the cells more rapidly. Blood is diverted from the gut and brain into skeletal muscles. This explains why many people don't think clearly under stress. Enzyme activity is diverted from its digestive tasks to those needed for energy production and increased respiratory capacity.

These functions are the body's natural way of being metabolically prepared for fight or flight. In prehistoric and ancient times, the energy produced was genuinely needed to battle the enemy or flee. However, modern society and the stress it produces infrequently presents a physical fight or flight situation. Human beings were designed to burn off the excess adrenaline as a result of the intense physical activity required for fighting or running away. Without that physical activity, adrenaline can take hours to metabolize and clear the system.

Suggestions for a Less Stressful Life

Follow these guidelines to make your life less stressful:

Be more tolerant of people and situations.

Be more patient—think before losing your cool.

Be a good listener—don't always have something to say and monopolize the conversation.

Develop meaningful relationships with those who you associate with, especially family.

Control aggressive behavior.

Work normal hours, improve your diet, and get sufficient sleep and rest.

Avoid stimulants, such as nicotine and caffeine, which will only exaggerate hyper, aggressive, anxious behavior.

Learn to accept what cannot be changed; work at changing only those things that can be changed.

Practice the exercises in the Serenity Prescription (next section) every day.

For many of us, managing stress, particularly emotional stress, is virtually impossible. As we discussed earlier, managing and controlling negative stress is essential to health and wellness. "Learn to relax" is an overused phrase that means nothing to most of us who frequently feel angry, anxious, upset, confused, frightened, and otherwise "out of control." Understanding what relaxation means and how to do it is key.

Although adrenaline is needed to effect physiological changes that provide us with that extra, temporary energy, it is a very powerful and dangerous oxidant substance, capable of severe free radical damage if not cleared from the system quickly. The extended presence of adrenaline in the system resulting from nonfight or flight stress keeps blood pressure dangerously elevated for hours. Vitamin C, needed for collagen production, immune support, and dozens of other functions, is severely depleted during periods of stress. The absence of collagen production, coupled with elevated blood pressure are weakening factors in cardiovascular disease. Additionally, the production of relaxing and painkilling neurotransmitter substances such as serotonin, dopamine, norepinephrine, enkephalins, and beta-endorphin cease or are downregulated to a minimal level. Last but not least, interrupted and incomplete digestion of food occurs as a result of enzyme activity shifting away from the digestive system.

The Serenity Prescription for Stress-Free Living

The recommendations, techniques, instructions, and suggestions below give most people a greater sense of serenity, calm, peacefulness, cheer, and mental clarity.

Breathe Right for Less Stress

The most critical thing we do—and the most unnoticed—is breathing. Chances are you don't breathe properly. Most of us breathe with our mouths open, typically taking short, shallow breaths that cause hyperventilation. This causes changes within the body such as feeling tense, nervous, and shaky, as well as dizziness and headaches. Chronic hyperventilation weakens breathing muscles (diaphragm and abdominals) over time, making it difficult to restore normal breathing patterns. Improved breathing can make you calm and improve you cardiovascular health.

Know if you are breathing correctly. Place one hand on your stomach and the other on your chest, palms down. If you are

> **The Breath Test**
> Count the number of normal breaths you take during a one-minute period. If it is more than fourteen, you are breathing too fast.

breathing right, the hand on your stomach will move outwards when you inhale and the hand on your chest will remain still. If the opposite happens, you are breathing incorrectly. Now—do it right, leaving your hands in place:

1. Exhale by pulling in your stomach, letting the air flow out through your nose (this not only improves breathing, it helps flatten the stomach).
2. Inhale slowly through your nose, letting your stomach expand outwards, without expanding your chest.
3. Repeat—counting three to five seconds for each inhale and three to five seconds for each exhale.
4. Practice this exercise for a minimum of five minutes each morning and evening, or more if you are feeling stressed. This can be practiced anywhere, at anytime. With regular practice this will become your predominant breathing style.

Release Physical Tension with Progressive Relaxation

Lie flat on your back on a semisoft surface, such as a carpeted floor or exercise mat, arms at your side, feet spread slightly apart. Tense each listed area of your body for five seconds. Then relax that area for five seconds. Notice how uncomfortable the "tense" sensation feels, then focus on how calm and relieving it feels when you relax each area.

Areas to be tensed and relaxed are the following (starting at the top and working your way down): ears, mouth, tongue, eyes, neck, shoulders, upper arms, forearms, hands, fingers, stomach, buttocks, thighs, knees, calves, ankles, arches, toes. Do this exercise in the morning and again in the evening!

Clear Your Mind

This exercise is extremely important for the cessation of negative, stressful, and depressing thoughts and thought patterns and that "brain clutter" feeling we all sometimes get. Find a completely quiet, dark place where you will be undisturbed.

Sit or lie down comfortably and close your eyes gently but completely. Imagine a bright-colored dot (pick your own color) shining between your eyes, just above eye level (in between the eyebrows). Focus on this dot until you can keep it in place. This takes practice! If you lose the focus, just bring it back again and again until you can hold it. Do not become upset if you cannot get it or hold it in the beginning. The duration of this exercise should be a minimum of five minutes. Do this exercise every morning and evening.

Rest Pleasurably

Here are some practical suggestions for "mellowing out." Put on loose, comfortable clothing and stretch out on your favorite "comfy" chair or couch. Read a good book, turn on your favorite music, watch a sad movie and have a good "cry," munch on a healthy snack, take a hot bath, and have no place to go. This is relaxation!

Sleep Properly

An adequate amount of sleep is required by all of us. During sleep the body repairs, heals, grows, and rejuvenates itself. It is a time period when stress is minimal, muscles relax, and heart rate and respiration slow down considerably. A poorly rested body is tense, incompletely repaired, lacking energy, and unable to think clearly. Follow these sleep basics:

- Get seven to eight hours of sleep nightly.
- Go to sleep at approximately the same time each night; this preserves your Circadian (day-night) rhythm.
- Sleep in a comfortable environment without the distractions of lights, TV, radio, and other disruptive noises and sights.

- Wear comfortable, temperature-appropriate clothes.
- Sleep on a quality pillow and mattress.

Develop a Positive Attitude

Research shows that negative emotions are toxic to the body. A bad attitude causes the body to produce excess amounts of stress-induced substances that initiate and perpetuate health-destroying effects on your body and suppress the ability to produce calming substances that are health promoting.

Notes

INTRODUCTION

1. American Heart Association, "1999 Heart and Stroke Statistical Update" (Dallas, Texas).
2. Centers for Disease Control, website: www.cdc.gov.
3. J. C. Paterson, *Canadian Medical Association Journal* 44 (1941): 114–20.

CHAPTER TWO

1. L. Zaret et al., *Yale University School of Medicine Heart Book* (New York: William Morrow and Company, 1992), 12.
2. Ibid., 21.
3. Anesthesia Clinics of North America, *Pathophysiology of Hypertension* 17, no. 3 (September 1999).
4. H. W. Wilmink et al., "Influence of Folic Acid on Postprandial Endothelial Dysfunction," *Arteriosclerosis, Thrombosis, and Vascular Biology* 20 (2000): 185–88.
5. S. Schroeder, "Non-Invasive Determination of Endothelial Mediated Vasodilation As a Screening Test for CAD: Pilot Study to Assess the Predictive Value in Comparison with Angina Pectoris, Exercise Electrocardiography and Myochardial Perfusion Imagery," *American Heart Journal* 138 (4 Pt. 1) (October 1999): 731–39.

6. M. Murray and J. Pizzorno, *Encyclopedia of Natural Medicine*, rev. 2d ed. (Rocklin, Calif.: Prima Publishing, 1998), 524.

7. W. B. Kannel, "Historic Perspectives on the Relative Contributions of Diastolic and Systolic Blood Pressure Elevation to Cardiovascular Risk Profile," *American Heart Journal* 138 (3 Pt. 2) (September 1999): 205–10.

8. F. Skrabal, J. Aubock, and H. Hortnagl, "Low Sodium? High Potassium Diet for Prevention of Hypertension, Probable Mechanisms of Action," *Lancet* 2 (1981): 895–900.

9. I. L. Rouse et al., "Vegetarian Diet and Blood Pressure," *Lancet* 2 (1983): 742–43.

10. T. Dyckner and P. Wester, "Effect of Magnesium on Blood Pressure," *British Medical Journal* 286 (1983): 1847–49.

11. L. Widman et al., "The Dose-Dependent Reduction in Blood Pressure Through Administration of Magnesium—a Double-Blind, Placebo-Controlled, Crossover Study," *American Journal of Hypertension* 6 (1993): 41–45.

12. J. Selhub et al., "Association Between Plasma Homocysteine Concentrations and Extracranial Carotid Artery Stenosis," *New England Journal of Medicine* 332 (1995): 286–91.

13. M. Gillmane et al., "Protective Effect of Fruits and Vegetables on Development of Stroke in Man," *Journal of the American Medical Association* 273 (1995): 1113–17.

14. S. C. Winter and N. R. M. Buist, "Cardiomyopathy in Childhood, Mitochondrial Dysfunction, and the Role of L-Carnitine," *American Heart Journal* 1139 (2 Pt. 3) (Suppl.) (2000): 563–69.

15. M. Murray and J. Pizzorno, *Encyclopedia of Natural Medicine*, rev. 2d ed. (Rocklin, Calif.: Prima Publishing, 1998), 101.

16. C. Pace-Asciak et al., "The Red Wine Phenolics Trans-Resveratrol and Quercetin Block Human Platelet Aggregation and Eicosanoid Synthesis: Implications for Protection Against Coronary Heart Disease," *Clinica Chimica hada* 235 (1995): 207–19.

17. M. Rath, "Eradicating Heart Disease," *Health Now* (1993):150.

18. E. Cranton, *Bypassing Bypass: The New Technique of Chelation Therapy*, rev. 2d ed. (Troutdale, Va.: Medex Publishers, 1994), 62.

19. W. Su et al., "Metabolism of Apo(A) and Apob100 of Lipoprotein (A) in Women: Effect of Post Menopausal Estrogen Replacement," *Journal of Clinical Endocrinology and Metabolism* 83, no. 9 (September 1998): 3267–76.

CHAPTER THREE

1. L. Zaret et al., *Yale University School of Medicine Heart Book* (New York: William Morrow and Company, 1992), 239.

2. M. Stampfer, "Vitamin E Consumption and the Risk of Coronary Artery Disease in Women," *New England Journal of Medicine* 328 (1993): 1444–49.

3. *Dorland's Illustrated Medical Dictionary*, 28th ed. (Philadelphia: W. B. Saunders Co., 1994).

4. A. L. Waterhouse, J. Shirley, and J. L. Donovan, "Antioxidants in Chocolate," *Lancet* 348, no. 9030 (1996): 834.

CHAPTER FIVE

1. I. Stone, *The Healing Factor, Vitamin C Against Disease* (New York: Grosset and Dunlap, 1972).

2. M. Rath and L. Pauling, "A Unified Theory of Human Cardiovascular Disease Leading the Way to the Abolition of This Disease as a Cause for Human Mortality," *Journal of Orthomolecular Medicine* 7 (1992): 5–15.

3. M. Rath, "Solution to the Puzzle of Human Evolution," *Journal of Orthomolecular Medicine* 7 (1992): 73–80.

4. J. E. Enstrom, E. Kanim, and M. A. Klein, "Vitamin C Intake and Mortality among a Sample of the United States Population," *Epidemiology* 3: 194–202.

5. P. C. Champe and R. A. Harvey, *Biochemistry* (Philadelphia: J. B. Lippincott, 1994), 219–330.

6. M. Rath, "Eradicating Heart Disease," *Health Now* (1993): 44.

CHAPTER SIX

1. D. Steinberg, "Beyond Cholesterol: Modifications of Low-Density Lipoprotein that Increase Its Atherogenicity," *New England Journal of Medicine* 320, no. 14 (1989): 915–24.
2. J. Regnstrim, "Susceptibility to Low-Density Lipoprotein Oxidation and Coronary Atherosclerosis in Man," *Lancet* 339 (1992): 1183–86.
3. S. Vallance, "Relationships Between Ascorbic Acid and Serum Proteins of the Immune System," *British Medical Journal* 2 (1977): 437–38.

CHAPTER SEVEN

1. R. A. Passwater, *FAQ's—All About Pycnogenol* (Garden City Park, N.Y.: Avery Publishing Group, 1998).
2. J. Challem, "Types of Free Radicals and Antioxidants," *The Nutrition Reporter* 7, no. 12 (1996): 1–2.
3. W. Harris, *Carcinogenesis* 15 (1992): 636–40.
4. R. H. Prior and G. Cao. "Total Antioxidant Capacity of Fruits," *Journal of Agriculture and Food Chemistry* 44 (1996): 701–5.
5. R. Prior and G. Cao, "Antioxidant Capacity and Polyphenolic Components of Teas: Implications for Altering in Vivo Antioxidant Status," *P.S.E.B.M.* (1999): 220, 255–61.
6. R. Prior et al., "Increases in Human Plasma Antioxidant Capacity after Consumption of Controlled Diets High in Fruit and Vegetables," *American Journal of Clinical Nutrition* 68 (1998): 1081–87.
7. I. K. Sledsewskaja et al., "Wobenzyme Administration in Patients after Myochardial Infarction. Oral Enzyme Therapy, Compendium of Results from Clinical Studies with Oral Enzyme Therapy (paper presented at 2d Russian Symposium, St. Petersburg, Russia, 1996), 90–92.

CHAPTER EIGHT

1. M. Rath, "Eradicating Heart Disease," *Health Now* (1993): 23.
2. Ibid., p. 48.

3. M. Rath, "Binding of Lipoproteins," *1991a, Trieu vn* (1991).

4. N. J. Wald et al., "Homocysteine and Ischemic Heart Disease: Results of a Prospective Study with Implications Regarding Prevention," *Archives of Internal Medicine* 158 (1998): 862–7.

5. J. Selhub et al., "Association between Plasma Homocysteine Concentrations and Extracranial Carotid Artery Stenosis," *New England Journal of Medicine* 332 (1995): 286–91.

6. P. M. Gallagher et al., "Homocysteine and the Risk of Premature Coronary Artery Disease. Evidence for a Common Gene Mutation," *Circulation* 94, no. 9 (1 November 1996): 2154–58.

7. E. B. Rimm et al., "Folate and Vitamin B_6 from Diet and Supplements in Relation to Risk of Coronary Heart Disease among Women," *Journal of the American Medical Association* 279 (1998): 359–64.

8. L. Leonhard, "Homocysteine and Cardiovascular Health," *Vitamin Research News* (September 1998), 1–4.

9. O. Lindberg et al., *Journal of the American Geriatric Society* 45, no. 4 (April 1997): 407–12.

10. G. M. Reaven, *Physiological Reviews* 75, no. 3 (1995): 473–75.

11. A. P. Simopoulos, "Is Insulin Resistance Influenced by Dietary Linoleic Acid and Trans-Fatty Acids?" *Free Radical Biology and Medicine* 17, no. 4 (1994): 367–72.

12. *Total Health* 22, no. 3: 2–3.

13. R. Ross, "Atherosclerosis—An Inflammatory Disease," *New England Journal of Medicine* 340 (1999): 115–26.

14. V. Foster, *The Vulnerable Atherosclerotic Plaque: Understanding, Identification, and Modification* (Armonk, N.Y.: Futura Publishing Co., 1999).

15. P. Ridker, and C. Hennekens, "C-Reactive Protein and Other Markers of Inflammation in the Prediction of Cardiovascular Disease in Women," *New England Journal of Medicine* 342 (2000): 36.

16. P. Ridker et al., "Prospective Studies on C-Reactive Protein as a Risk Factor for Cardiovascular Disease," *Investigative Medicine* 46 (1998): 391.

17. E. Shattuck Braunwauld, "Cardiovascular Medicine at the Turn of the Millennium: Triumphs, Concerns, and Opportunities," *New England Journal of Medicine* 337 (1997): 1360–69.

18. A. J. Ahmed, "Systemic Enzymes: No More Shooting Rubber Bands at the Moon," *Total Health* 22 (2000): 54.

19. L. Stryker, *Biochemistry*, 3d ed. (New York: W. H. Freeman and Company, 1988), 249.

20. E. Ernst, "Fibrinogen: An Important Risk Factor for Athero-thrombotic Diseases," *Annals of Medicine* 26 (1994): 15–22.

21. G. B. Rosito, *Cardiology Clinics* 14, no. 2 (May 1996): 239–50.

22. L. Stryker, *Biochemistry*, 3d ed.(New York: W. H. Freeman and Company, 1988), 252.

23. M. Murray and J. Pizzorno, *Encyclopedia of Natural Medicine*, rev. 2d ed. (Rocklin, Calif.: Prima Publishing, 1998), 96.

24. Arfenist Lam et al., "Investigation of Possible Mechanisms of Pyridoxal 5-Phosphate Inhibition of Platelet Reactions," *Thrombosis Research* 20 (1980): 633–45.

25. A. Sewrmet et al., "Effect of Oral Pyridoxine Hydrochloride Supplementation on In Vitro Platelet Sensitivity to Different Antagonists," *Arzneim Forsch* 45 (1995): 19–21.

26. C. Pace-Asciak et al., "The Red Wine Phenolics Trans-Resveratrol and Quercetin Block Human Platelet Aggregation and Eicosanoid Synthesis: Implications for Protection Against Coronary Heart Disease," *Clinica Chimica hada* 235 (1995): 207–19.

CHAPTER NINE

1. J. Yudkin, I. Edelman, and L. Hough, eds., *Sugar; Chemical, Biological and Nutritional Aspects of Sucrose* (Hartford: Daniel Davey, 1971).

2. R. A. Passwater, *Lipoic Acid: The Metabolic Antioxidant* (New Canaan, Conn.: Keats Publishing, 1995), 29.

3. Ibid.

4. A. Sharma et al., "Vitamin E Protects Against Free Radical Damage in Diabetes Evaluation of Oxidative Stress Before and After Control of Glycemia and After Vitamin E Supplementation in Diabetic Patients," *Metabolic Clinical Experiments* 49 (2000): 160–62.

5. A. Reddi et al., "Biotin Supplementation Improves Glucose and Insulin Tolerance in Genetically Diabetic KK Mice," *Life Sciences* 42 (1988): 1323–30.

6. U.S. Department of Health and Human Services, *The Surgeon General's Report on Nutrition and Health*, PHS publication No. 88-50210 (1988).

7. E. N. Siguel, *Essential Fatty Acids in Health and Disease* (Brookline, Mass.: Nutrek Press, 1994), 171.

8. D. S. Siscovick and T. E. Raghunathan, "Dietary Intake and Cell Membrane Levels of Long Chain N-3 Polyunsaturated Fatty Acids and the Risk of Primary Cardiac Arrest," *Journal of the American Medical Association* 274, no. 17 (1 November 1995).

9. J. A. Conquer and B. Holub, "Supplementation with an Algae Source of Docosahexaenoic Acid Increases (N-3) Fatty Acid Status Alters Selected Risk Factors for Heart Disease in Vegetarian Subjects," *Journal of Nutrition* 126 (1996): 3032–39.

10. E. N. Siguel, *Essential Fatty Acids in Health and Disease* (Brookline, Mass.: Nutrek Press, 1994), 171.

11. Ibid., p. 22.

12. W. S. Harris et al., "N-3 Fatty Acids and Urinary Excretion of Nitric Oxide Metabolites in Humans," *American Journal of Clinical Nutrition* 65 (1997): 459–64.

13. M. Fisher, K. S. Upchurch, and J. J. Hoogasian, "Effects of Dietary Fish Oil Supplementation on Polymorphonuclear Leukocyte Inflammatory Potential," *Inflammation* 10, no. 4 (1986): 387–92.

14. M. L. Daviglus, "Fish Consumption and the 30-Year Risk of Myochardial Infarction," *New England Journal of Medicine* 336 (1977): 1046–53.

15. J. Dyerberg, H. O. Bang, and O. Aagahard, "Small Is Beautiful: Alpha Linolenic Acid and Eicosapentaenoic Acid in Man," *Lancet* (21 May 1983): 1169.

16. K. Radack, C. Deck, and C. Huster, "Dietary Supplementation with Low-Dose Fish Oils Lowers Fibrinogen Levels: A Randomized, Double Blind Controlled Study," *Annals of Internal Medicine* 11, no. 9 (1989): 757–58.

17. A. G. Leaf, E. Billman, and H. Hallaq, "Prevention of Ischemia-Induced Ventricular Fibrillation by Omega-3 Fatty Acids," *Proceedings of the National Academy of Science* 91 (1994): 4427–30.

CHAPTER TEN

1. K. A. Matthews and S. G. Haynes, "Type A Behavior Pattern and Coronary Disease Risk," *American Journal of Epidemiology* 123 (1986): 923–60.

2. U. Lundberg et al., "Type A Behavior in Healthy Males and Females as Related to Physiologic Reactivity and Blood Lipids," *Psychosomatic Medicine* 51 (1989): 113–22.

3. M. M. Muller et al., "The Relationship between Habitual Anger Coping Style and Serum Lipid and Lipoprotein Concentrations, *Biological Psychology* 41 (1995): 69–81.

4. L. D. Kubzansky et al., "Is Worrying Bad for Your Heart, a Prospective Study of Worry and Coronary Heart Disease in Normative Aging Study," *Circulation* 95 (1997): 818–24.

5. W. Raab, "Cardiotoxic Effects of Emotional, Socioeconomic, and Environmental Stresses," *Myocardiology* 1 (1970): 707–13.

6. J. G. Henrotte, "Type A Behavior and Magnesium Metabolism," *Magnesium* 5 (1986): 201–10.

7. L. Zaret et al., *Yale University School of Medicine Heart Book* (New York: William Morrow and Company, 1992), 30, 72.

8. Ibid., p. 73.

9. Ibid.

10. J. E. Enstrom, L. E. Kanim, and M. A. Klein, "Vitamin C Intake and Mortality among a Sample of the United States Population," *Epidemiology* 3: 194–202.

CHAPTER ELEVEN

1. E. E. Snell, E. L. Thatum, and W. H. Peterson, *Journal of Bacteriology* 33 (1937): 207.

CHAPTER TWELVE

1. R. A. Passwater, *Lipoic Acid: The Metabolic Antioxidant* (New Canaan, Conn.: Keats Publishing, Inc., 1995), 16, 23.
2. Ibid.
3. L. Packer, "Free Radical Biology and Medicine," 19, no. 2 (1995): 227–50.
4. R. Kirchoff et al., "Increase in Choleresis by Means of Artichoke Extract," *Phytomedicine* 1 (1994): 107–15.
5. R. Gebhardt, "Artichoke Extract. in Vitro Proof of Cholesterol Biosynthesis Inhibition," *Medwelt* 46 (1995): 348–50.
6. K. Kraft, "Artichoke Extract—Recent Findings Reflecting Effects on Lipid Metabolism, Liver, and Gastrointestinal Tracts," *Phytomedicine* 4 (1997): 369–78.
7. D. Morris, "Serum Carotenoids and Coronary Artery Disease," *Journal of the American Medical Association* 272 (1994): 1439–41.
8. E. S. Ford and W. H. Giles, "Serum Vitamins, Carotenoids, and Angina Pectoris," *Annals of Epidemiology* 10 (2000): 106–16.
9. O. M. Panasenko et al., "Interaction of Peroxynitrite with Carotenoids in Human Low-Density Lipoproteins," *Archives of Biochemical Biophysics* 272 (2000): 302–5.
10. Arfenist Lam et al., "Investigation of Possible Mechanisms of Pyridoxal 5-Phosphate Inhibition of Platelet Reactions," *Thrombosis Research* 202.

11. A. Sewrmet et al., "Effect of Oral Pyridoxine Hydrochloride Supplementation on In Vitro Platelet Sensitivity to Different Antagonists," *Arzneim Forsch* 45 (1995): 19–21.

12. A. Reddi et al., "Biotin Supplementation Improves Glucose and Insulin Tolerance in Genetically Diabetic KK Mice," *Life Sciences* 42 (1988): 1323–30.

13. A. Raman, A. Lau, and C. Lau, *Phytomedicine* 7, no. 4 (1996): 349–62.

14. T. Kawada et al., "Effects of Capsaicin on Lipid Metabolism in Rats Fed a High Fat Diet," *Journal of Nutrition* 116 (1986): 1272–78.

15. S. Visudhipan et al., "The Relationship between High Fibrinolytic Activity and Daily Capsicum Ingestion in Thais," *American Journal of Clinical Nutrition* 35 (1982): 1452–58.

16. G. Fraser et al., "The Effect of Various Vegetable Substances on Serum Cholesterol," *American Journal of Clinical Nutrition* 34 (1981): 1272–77.

17. C. A. Rice-Evans, N. Miller, and G. Paganga, "Structure—Antioxidant Activity Relationships of Flavonoids and Phenolic Acids," *Free Radical Biology and Medicine* 20, no.7 (1996): 933–56.

18. R. A. Anderson and R. S. Koslovsky, "Chromium Intake, Absorption, and Excretion of Subjects Consuming Self-Elected Diets," *American Journal of Clinical Nutrition* 41 (1985): 1177–83.

19. R. A. Anderson, "Chromium, Glucose Intolerance, and Diabetes," *Journal of the American College of Nutrition* 17 (1998): 548–55.

20. R. A. Anderson et al., *Diabetes* 46, no.11 (1997): 1786–91.

21. N. Mirsky, *Arefuah* 132, no. 2 (1997): 133–6.

22. E. G. Offenbacher et al., *Diabetes* 29 (1980): 919.

23. C. Morisco, *Journal of Clinical Investigation* 71 (1993): S134–S136.

24. W. V. Judy, W. W. Stodghill, and K. Folkers, "Myochardial Preservation by Therapy with Coenzyme Q10 During Heart Surgery," *Journal of Clinical Investigation* 71 (1993): S155–S161.

25. S. Segal and J. Foley, *Journal of Clinical Investigation* 37 (1958): 719–35.

26. H. G. Zimmer and H. Ibel, "Ribose Accelerates Repletion of the ATP Pool During Recovery from Reversible Ischemia of the Rat Myochardium," *Journal of Molecular and Cellular Cardiology* 16 (1984): 863–66.

27. Y. Hellsten-Westing et al., "Decreased Resting Levels of Adenine Nucleotides in Human Skeletal Muscle after High Intensity Training," *Journal of Applied Physiology* 74, no. 5 (1993): 2523–28.

28. H. G. Zimmer et al., "Ribose Intervention in the Cardiac Pentose Phosphate Pathway Is Not Species Specific," *Science* 223 (1984): 712–14.

29. E. Gerlach, *Pfleugers Archives* 376 (1978): 223.

30. J. Budwig, *Flax Oil as a True Aid Against Arthritis, Heart Infarction, Cancer, and Other Disease* (Vancouver: Apple Publishing, 1992).

31. E. B. Rimm et al., "Folate and Vitamin B_6 from Diet and Supplements in Relation to Risk of Coronary Heart Disease among Women," *Journal of the American Medical Association* 279 (1998): 359–64.

32. L. Leonhard, "Homocysteine and Cardiovascular Health," *Vitamin Research News* (September 1998): 1–4.

33. R. M. Russell, "A Minimum of 13,500 Deaths from Coronary Artery Disease Could Be Prevented by Increasing Folate Intake to Reduce Homocysteine Levels," *Journal of the American Medical Association* 275 (1996): 1828–29.

34. A. K. Jain, *American Journal of Medicine* 94 (1993): 632.

35. N. Ide and B. H. S. Lau, "A-Allylcysteine Attenuates Oxidative Stress in Endothelial Cells," *Drug Development and Industrial Pharmacy* 25, no. 5 (1999): 619–24.

36. N. Ide et al., "Antioxidant Effects of Fructosyl Arginine, a Maillhard Reaction Product in Aged Garlic Extract," *Journal of Nutritional Biochemistry* 10 (1999): 372–76.

37. F. G. McMahon et al., *Pharmacotherapy* 13 , no. 4 (1993): 406.

38. S. Kasuga et al., "Effect of Aged Garlic Extract (AGE) on Hyperglycemia Induced by Immobilization Stress in Mice," *Nippon Yakurigaku Zasshi* 114, no. 3 (1999): 191–97.

39. N. Ide and B. H. Lau, "Aged Garlic Extract Attenuates Intracellular Oxidative Stress," *PhytoMedicine* 6, no. 2 (1999): 125–31.

40. M. Murray, *The Healing Power of Herbs: The Enlightened Persons Guide to the Wonders of Medicinal Plants* (Rocklin, Calif.: Prima Publishing, 1992), 118–22.

41. K. Wesnes et al., *Human Psychopharmacology: Clinical and Experimental* 2 (1987): 159.

42. P. Jung et al., *Arzneim-Forsch* 40, no. 5 (1990): 589.

43. D. Bagchi et al., "Oxygen Free Radical Scavenging Abilities of Vitamin C and E and a Grapeseed Proanthocyanidin Extract In Vitro," *Research Communications in Molecular Pathology and Pharmacology*, 95 (1997): 179–89.

44. J. Masquelier, M. C. Dumon, and J. Dumas, "Stabilization of Collagen by Procyanidolic Oligomers," *Acta Therap* 7 (1981): 101–5.

45. Food Research Laboratories, "Prophylactic Functions of Tea Polyphenols" (Japan: Mutsui Norin Co., Ltd., 1998).

46. S. J. Miura et al., "The Inhibitory Effects of Tea Polyphenols (Flavan-3-ol Derivatives) on Cu+2 Mediated Oxidative Modification of Low Density Lipoprotein," *Biological and Pharmaceutical Bulletin* 17, no. 12 (1994): 1567–72.

47. I. Ikeda et al., "Tea Catechins Decrease Micellar Solubility and Intestinal Absorption of Cholesterol in Rats," *Biochemia et Biophysica Acta* 1127 (1992): 141–46.

48. D. F. Fitzpatrick et al., "Endothelium Dependent Relaxation Caused by Various Plant Extracts," *Journal of Cardiovascular Pharmacology* (1995).

49. C. A. Rice-Evans, N. Miller, and G. Paganga, "Structure—Antioxidant Activity Relationships of Flavonoids and Phenolic Acids," *Free Radical Biology and Medicine* 20, no. 7 (1996): 933–56.

50. M. Ali et al., "A Potent Thromboxane Formation Inhibitor in Green Tea Leaves," *Prostaglandins, Leukotrienes, and Essential Fatty Acids* 40, no. 4 (1990): 281–83.

51. G. V. Satyavati, *Plants and Traditional Medicine* 5 (1982): 47–82.

52. ———, "Guggulipid, A Promising Hypolipaedemic Agent from Gum Guggul," *Econ Plant Medical Research* 5 (1991): 47–82.

53. M. T. Murray, *The Healing Power of Herbs, The Enlightened Persons Guide to the Wonders of Medicinal Plants* (Rocklin, Calif.: Prima Publishing, 1992), 203–9.

54. Y. Nasa et al., "Protective Effect of Crataegus Extract on the Cardiac Mechanical Dysfunction in Isolated Perfused Rat Heart," *Arzneimittel-Forschung* 43 (1993): 945–49.

55. M. Gabor, "Pharmacologic Effects of Flavonoids on Blood Vessels," *Angiologica* 9 (1972): 355–74.

56. Ibid.

57. V. W. Rewerski et al., *Arzneimittel-Forschung* 17 (1967): 490–91.

58. H. Leuchtgens, *Fortschchitte Medizin* 111 (1993): 352–54.

59. M. A. Creager et al., "L-Arginine Improves Endothelium Dependent Vasodilation in Hypocholesterolimic Humans," *Journal of Clinical Investigation* 90 (1992): 1248–53.

60. S. Mohta, D. J. Stewart, and D. J. Levy, "The Hypotensive Effect of L-Arginine Is Associated with Increased Expired Nitric Oxide in Humans," *Chest* 109, no. 6 (1996): 1550–56.

61. R. Ambrect et al., "Correction of Endothelial Dysfunction in Chronic Heart Failure: Additional Effects of Exercise Training and Oral L-Arginine Supplementation," *Journal of the American College of Cardiology* 35, no. 3 (2000): 706–13.

62. I. B. Fritz, "Action of Carnitine on Long Chain Fatty Acid Oxidation by Liver," *American Journal of Physiology* 197 (1959): 297–304.

63. L. H. Opie, "Role of Carnitine in Fatty Acid Metabolism of Normal and Ischemic Myochardium," *American Heart Journal* 97 (1979): 375–88.

64. E. R. Braverman, *The Healing Nutrients Within* (New Canaan, Conn.: Keats Publishing, 1997), 140–43.

65. H. A. Schroeder, "Losses of Vitamins and Trace Minerals Resulting from Processing and Preservation of Foods," *American Journal of Clinical Nutrition* 24 (1971): 562–73.

66. J. G. Henrotte, "Type A Behavior and Magnesium Metabolism," *Magnesium* 5 (1986): 201–10, 12.

67. B. Altura, "Cardiovascular Risk Factors and Magnesium," *Magnesium Trace Elements* 10 (1991–92): 182–92.

68. A. Bajusz and E. Selye, "The Chemical Prevention of Cardiac Necroses Following Occlusion of Coronary Vessels," *Canadian Medical Association Journal* 82 (1960): 212–13.

69. A. Gaby, *Magnesium: How an Important Mineral Helps Prevent Heart Attacks and Relieve Stress* (New Canaan, Conn.: Keats Publishing, 1994), 19–23.

70. K. Satake et al., "Relation between Severity of Magnesium Deficiency and Frequency of Anginal Attacks in Men with Variant Angina," *Journal of the American College of Cardiology* 28, no. 4 (1996): 897–902.

71. Cardinal Nutrition, website: www.cardinalnutrition.com.

72. C. Weatherby and L. Gordon, *The Arthritis Bible* (Rochester, Vt.: Healing Arts Press, 1999), 50.

73. P. L. Canner et al., "Fifteen Year Mortality in Coronary Drug Project Patients, Long-Term Benefit with Niacin," *Journal of the American College of Cardiology* 8 (1986): 1245–55.

74. D. R. Illingworth et al., "Comparative Effects of Lovasthatin and Niacin in Primary Hypercholesterolimia," *Archives of Internal Medicine* 154 (1994): 1586–95.

75. P. J. Jones et al., "Dietary Phytosterols as Cholesterol Lowering Agents in Humans," *Canadian Journal of Physiological Pharmacology* 75 (1997): 217–27.

76. X. Pelletier et al., "A Diet Moderately Enriched in Phytosterols Lowers Plasma Cholesterol Concentrations in Normocholes-

terolimic Humans," *Annals of Nutritional Metabolism* 39 (1995): 291–95.

77. P. Kopp, "Resveratrol, a Phytoestrogen Found in Red Wine. A Possible Explanation for the Conundrum of the 'French Paradox?'" *European Journal of Endocrinology* 138 (1998): 619–20.

78. L. Stanley et al., "Potential Explanations for the French Paradox," *Nutritional Research* 19 (1999): 3–15.

79. C. Pace-Asciak et al., "The Red Wine Phenolics Trans-Resveratrol and Quercetin Block Human Platelet Aggregation and Eicosanoid Synthesis: Implications for Protection Against Coronary Heart Disease," *Clinica Chimica hada* 235 (1995): 207–19.

80. Ibid.

81. Ibid.

82. H. Arichi et al., "Effects of Stilbene Components of the Roots of Polygonum Cuspidatum Sieb. et Zucc. on Lipid Metabolism," *Chemistry and Pharmacological Bulletin* 30 (1982): 1766–70.

83. C. Chen and C. Pace-Asciak, "Vasorelaxing Activity of Resveratrol and Quercetin in Isolated Rat Aorta," *General Pharmaceuticals* 27 (1996): 363–66.

84. S. Chanvitayanpongs et al., "Amelioration of Oxidative Stress by Antioxidant and Resveratrol in PCI2 Cells," *Neuroreport* 8 (1997): 1499–1502.

85. A. Leung and Z. Mo, "Protective Effects of Polydatin, an Active Compound from Polygonum Cuspida Turn, on Cerebral Ischemia Damage in Rats," *Chinese Pharmaceutical Bulletin* 12 (1996): 128–29.

86. S. V. Nigdika et al., "Consumption of Red Wine Polyphenols Reduces the Susceptibility of Low-Density Lipoproteins to Oxidation In Vivo," *American Journal of Clinical Nutrition* 68 (1998): 258–65.

87. F. Frankel et al., "Inhibition of Human LDL Oxidation by Resveratrol," *Lancet* 341 (1993): 1103–4.

88. V. Badmaev and M. Majeed, *Alternative Therapies* 2, no. 4 (1996): 59–65.

89. F. Kok et al., "Decreased Selenium Levels in Acute Myochardial Infarction," *Journal of the American Medical Association* 261 (1989): 1161–64.

90. Q. H. Meng et al., "Incorporation of Esterified Soybean Isoflavones with Antioxidant Activity into Low-Density Lipoprotein," *Biochem et Biophys Acta Mol Cell Biol Lipids* 1438, no. 3 (1999): 369–76.

91. J. R. Crouse III et al., "A Randomized Trial Comparing the Effect of Casein with That of Soy Protein Containing Varying Amounts of Isoflavones on Plasma Concentrations of Lipids and Lipoproteins," *Archives of Internal Medicine* 159 (1999): 2070–76.

92. A. Ramamoorthy and S. Premakumari, Department of Food Science and Nutrition, Avinashilingam Institute for Home Science (Deemed University) Coimbatore-641 043, India, "Effect of Supplementation of Spirulina on Hypercholesterolemic Patients," *Journal of Food Science Technology* 33, no. 2 (1996): 124–12.

93. M. S. Miranda et al., "Antioxidant Activity of the Microalga Spirulina Maxima," *Brazilian Journal of Medical and Biological Research* 31, no. 8 (August 1998): 1075–79.

94. C. Romay et al., "Antioxidant and Anti-Inflammatory Properties of C-Phycocyanin from Blue-Green Algae," *Inflammation Research* 47 (1998): 36–41.

95. M. Paredes et al., "Effects of Dietary Spirulina Maxima on Endothelium Dependent Vasomotor Responses of Rat Aortic Rings," *Life Sciences* 61, no. 15 (1997): 211–19.

96. C. Furnsinn et al., *International Journal of Obesity and Related Metabolic Disorders* 19 (1995): 458–63.

97. B. F. Arland et al., *Journal of the American Dietetic Association* 94 (1994): 891–894.

98. S. Goodman, *Vitamin C: The Master Nutrient* (New Canaan, Conn.: Keats Publishing, 1991).

99. E. Niki, "Interaction of Ascorbate and A-Tocopherol. Third Conference on Vitamin C," *Annals of New York Academy of Sciences* 498 (1998).

100. M. K. Bartlett, C. M. Jones, and A. E. Ryan, "Vitamin C and Wound Healing. II. Ascorbic Acid Content and Tensile Strength of Healing Wounds in Human Beings," *New England Journal of Medicine* 226 (1942): 474–81.

101. A. J. Verlangieri, B. A. Chardin, and M. Bush, "The Interaction of Aortic Glycosaminoglycans and Insulin Endothelial Permeability in Cholesterol Induced Rabbit," *Atherogenesis* 224 (1985), reported by S. Goodman in *Vitamin C: The Master Nutrient* (New Canaan, Conn.: Keats Publishing, 1991).

102. A. J. Verlangieri, "The Role of Vitamin C in Diabetic and Non Diabetic Atherosclerosis," *Bulletin, Bureau of Pharmaceutical Services, University of Mississippi* 21 (1985): 223.

103. ———, "Effects of Vitamin C and Vitamin E on Induced Primate," *Atherosclerosis* 230 (1989).

104. J. M. Rogoff et al., "Vitamin C and Insulin Action," *Pennsylvania Medical Journal* 47 (1944): 579–82.

105. A. C. Chan, "Partners in Defense, Vitamin E and Vitamin C," *Canadian Journal of Physiological Pharmacology* 71, no. 9 (1993): b725–b731.

106. M. O'Keefe et al., American Chemical Society meeting, New Orleans, August 1999.

107. G. M. Reaven et al., "Effect of Dietary Antioxidant Combinations in Humans, Protection of LDL by Vitamin E but Not by Beta-Carotene," *Arteriosclerosis Thrombosis* 13, no. 4 (1993): 590–600.

108. E. Kronhousen et al., "Formula for Life: The Anti-Oxidant, Free Radical Detoxification Program" 9 (1989): 108–13; and A. M. Ochsner et al., *Journal of the American Medical Association* 144 (1950): 831–34.

109. M. J. Stampfer et al., "Vitamin E Consumption and the Risk of Coronary Disease in Women," *New England Journal of Medicine* 328 (1993): 1444–48.

110. E. B. Rimm, "Vitamin E Consumption and the Risk of Coronary Heart Disease in Men," *New England Journal of Medicine* 328 (1993): 1450–55.

111. A. M. Jenkinson et al., "The Effect of Increased Intakes of Polyunsaturated Fatty Acids and Vitamin E on DNA Damage in Human Lymphocytes," *FASEB Journal* 13 (1999): 2138–42.

112. M. Steiner, "Vitamin E: More Than an Antioxidant," *Clinical Cardiology* 16 (Suppl.1) (1993): 116–18.

113. H. Hodis et al., "Serial Coronary Angiographic Evidence that Antioxidant Vitamin Intake Reduces Progression of Coronary Artery Atherosclerosis," *Journal of the American Medical Association* 273 (1995): 1849–54.

114. N. A. Stephens et al., "Vitamin E Supplementation in Coronary Disease Patients," *Lancet* 347 (1996): 781–86.

115. M. Murray and J. Pizzorno, *Encyclopedia of Natural Medicine*, rev. 2d ed. (Rocklin, Calif.: Prima Publishing, 1998), 75.

116. P. Leskovar, "AIDS: Neuartige Therapiekonzepte," *Deutsche Zeitschrift Onkologie* (1990).

117. I. K. Sledsewskaja et al., "Wobenzym Administration in Patients after Myochardial Infarction. Oral Enzyme Therapy. Compendium of Results from Clinical Studies with Oral Enzyme Therapy" (paper presented at 2d Russian Symposium, St. Petersburg, Russia, 1996).

Glossary

Aerobic: Requiring oxygen for respiration.

Aggregation: Clumping or sticking together.

Alkaloids: Specific nitrogen-containing phytonutrients (*phyto* = plant) that have health-promoting abilities.

Amino acids: The building blocks of protein, nitrogen-containing nutrients, sometimes found freely in foods or formed from dietary proteins, and then converted into metabolic "building" proteins.

Anaerobic: Not requiring oxygen for respiration.

Antioxidant: Substance that protects other substances from free radical damage and oxidation.

Arteriosclerosis: Stiffening and hardening of the arteries that leads to high blood pressure and cardiovascular accidents.

Atherogenic: A substance or metabolite, or physiological action that causes atherogenesis, the initiation of the formation of atherosclerotic plaques.

Atherosclerosis: Buildup of fatty deposits, called plaques, on artery walls that narrows blood vessels.

Beta-carotene: An orange-colored, vitamin-like nutrient found in foods that is converted into vitamin A by the liver and functions as an antioxidant.

Bioflavonoids: A group of naturally occurring phytonutrients in food that are pigments (coloring substances) and powerful antioxidants.

CAD: Commonly referred to as coronary artery disease, of which there are many types.

Cardiotonic: Any nutrient that increases the efficiency of the heart.

Carotenoids: Phytonutrients, yellow to red plant pigments that are antioxidants.

Carotid arteries: The two major arteries that run alongside the neck and carry the blood supply to the brain.

Catechins: Phytonutrients, a term used to mean the polyphenols found in green tea, that allow themselves to be oxidized (biologically rusted) instead of more essential molecules.

Chelation: Means "clawing," a process in which a body substance chelates—attaches—itself to another substance, transporting it through the body, or carrying it out of the body.

Chlorophyll: The natural green pigment substance found in all green plants.

Co-enzyme: A biological helper substance that allows other nutrients to perform their tasks but does not get changed or used in the process.

Collagen: A primary protein that is the main component of connective tissues.

CVA: Commonly referred to as cardiovascular accidents—stroke and heart attack.

DNA: Deoxyribonucleic acid. Genetic code material.

Enzymes: Biological protein substances that function as helpers to allow chemical reactions to take place without being chemically changed themselves.

Epidemiological: A study of the causes and frequency of a disease in a defined population group.

Etiology: The causative factors of symptoms, diseases, conditions, or syndromes.

Free radicals: Atoms or molecules that have one electron missing that steal an electron from a healthy molecule.

Glucose: Nature's simplest form of sugar, and the body's main fuel.

Insulin: A hormone produced by the pancreas that regulates blood sugar levels.

Lesion: A break or discontinuation of tissue that impairs its function.

Leukotrienes: Eicosanoids produced from fatty acids that cause inflammatory conditions and bronchial spasms.

Lipoprotein (a): An adhesive "sticky" version of LDL (low-density lipoprotein) cholesterol that readily attaches to artery walls.

Metabolic: Referring to metabolism, which is the sum of all building-up processes in the body (anabolism), and all breakdown processes in the body (catabolism).

Metabolite: Any substance produced by metabolism or a metabolic process.

Microgram: 1/1000th of a milligram.

Micromole: A laboratory unit of measure.

Mutation: A change, generally negative, in the genetic makeup of a cell.

Neurotransmitters: Chemical substances responsible for transmission of chemical signals in the brain.

Orthomolecular: Term coined by Nobel laureate Linus Pauling, meaning "right" molecule. Refers to the use of correct natural substances to balance the body's molecules and promote health.

Oxidation: Biological "rusting" when oxygen attaches to and destroys cells.

Pathogen: Any invading organisms, such as bacteria, viruses, and parasites that are dangerous to human health.

Photosynthesis: A chemical process occurring in plants, where plants capture light energy from the sun, converting it with help from chlorophyll and carbon dioxide into food energy and oxygen.

Phytonutrients: *Phyto* = plant. Natural nutrient substances found in plants.

Plasma: The fluid portion of the blood in which the components are suspended.

Prostaglandins: Localized hormonelike substances produced from essential fatty acids that regulate body functions.

Proteolytic: A substance that breaks down proteins.

RNA: Ribonucleic acid. Translates DNA codes into metabolic (building block) proteins.

Serotonin: A neurotransmitter substance that has a calming effect, and signals the body that it is no longer hungry.

Stenosis: In cardiovascular disease, the narrowing of an artery.

Synergistic: A substance that assists the beneficial activity of another substance, causing its own beneficial effect.

Thromboxane: An eicosanoid produced from arachadonic acid (AA) that is known to cause abnormal clotting of blood in arteries.

Toxins: A broad term referring to poisons that can cause death in humans and other living things.

Recommended Readings
and Resources

Bushkin, E., and G. Bushkin. *FAQ's—All About Green Food Supplements*. Garden City Park, N.Y.: Avery Publishing, 1999.

Challem, J., and V. Dolby. *Homocysteine: The Secret Killer*. New Canaan, Conn.: Keats Publishing, 1997.

———. *Homocysteine: The New Cholesterol*. New Canaan, Conn.: Keats Publishing, 1996.

Dorland's Illustrated Medical Dictionary. 28th ed. Philadelphia: W. B. Saunders Co., 1994.

Fischbach, F. A. *Manual of Laboratory & Diagnostic Tests*. 4th ed. Philadelphia: J. B. Lippincott Company, 1992.

Holt, S. *Soya for Health: The Definitive Medical Guide*. Larchmont, N.Y.: Mary Ann Liebert, Inc., 1996.

Lopez, D. A., Williams, R. M., Miehlke, K. *Enzymes: Fountain of Life*. Neville Press, 1994.

McCully K. S. *The Homocysteine Revolution*. New Canaan, Conn.: Keats Publishing, 1997.

Murray, M., and J. Pizzorno. *Encyclopedia of Natural Medicine*. Rev. 2d ed. Rocklin, Calif.: Prima Publishing, 1998.

Passwater, R. A. *Lipoic Acid: The Metabolic Antioxidant*. New Canaan, Conn.: Keats Publishing, Inc., 1995.

———. *FAQ's—All About Pycnogenol*. Garden City Park, N.Y.: Avery Publishing Group, 1998.

Rath, M. "Eradicating Heart Disease," *Health Now*. 1993.

Seibold, R. S. "Cereal Grass: What's In It For You." Lawrence, Kansas: Wilderness Community Education Foundation, Inc., 1990.

Siguel, E. N. *Essential Fatty Acids in Health and Disease*. Brookline, Mass.: Nutrek Press, 1994.

Stryker, L. *Biochemistry*. 3d ed. New York: W. H. Freeman and Company, 1988.

Ulene, A. *The Nutribase Nutrition Facts Desk Reference*. Garden City Park, N.Y.: Avery Publishing Group, 1995.

Zaret, L. et al. *Yale University School of Medicine Heart Book*, New York: William Morrow and Company, 1992.

INTERNET SITES

www.chardinalnutrition.com
A discussion of MSM (methylsulfonylmethane, an anti-inflammatory nutriceutical)

lonza.com
A discussion of carnitine

mdconsult.com
A discussion of health conditions and disorders

www.rath.nl
A discussion of heart disease and natural therapies

www.wheatgrass.com
A discussion of wheatgrass and other cereal grasses

www.americanheart.com
Sponsored by the American Heart Association

www.nlm.nih.gov/databases/freemedl.html
Medline (for medical journal abstracts)

Index